KW-043-827

CONTENTS

HOUSE OF LORDS

SESSION 1999–2000
6th REPORT

SELECT COMMITTEE ON SCIENCE AND TECHNOLOGY

Ordered to be printed
21 November 2000

LONDON : THE STATIONERY OFFICE
£15·50

HL Paper 123

Note

Written and oral evidence received by the Committee is published in two separate volumes (HL Paper 48 and HL Paper 118).

In the text of the Report:

Q refers to a question in oral evidence;
p refers to a page of written evidence printed in HL Paper 118; and
P refers to a page of written evidence printed in HL Paper 48.

SIXTH REPORT

---

21 November 2000

By the Select Committee appointed to consider Science and Technology.

Ordered to Report

COMPLEMENTARY AND ALTERNATIVE MEDICINE

SUMMARY

I. The use of complementary and alternative medicine (CAM) is widespread and increasing across the developed world. This raises significant issues of public health policy such as whether good structures of regulation to protect the public are in place; whether an evidence base has been accumulated and research is being carried out; whether there are adequate information sources on the subject; whether the practitioner's training is adequate and what the prospects are for NHS provision of these treatments. It was the need to consider these issues that prompted this Inquiry (Chapter 1).

II. CAM includes a large range of therapies. Some offer complete systems of assessment and treatment, others complement conventional treatment with various supportive techniques. Some have well-developed regulatory structures, others are fragmented professions with little interdisciplinary agreement about regulation. A few have begun to build an evidence base, most have not. The Committee have proposed three groups of CAM therapies. Group 1 includes the most organised professions; Group 2 contains those therapies that most clearly complement conventional medicine. While the question of efficacy was not included in our initial terms of reference, in the absence of a credible evidence base it is our opinion that the therapies listed in our Group 3 cannot be supported unless and until convincing research evidence of efficacy, based upon the results of well designed trials, can be produced. Such evidence must be capable of showing that the effects of any therapeutic discipline are superior to those of the placebo effect (see paras 3.19 – 3.34). It is our view that for those therapies in our Group 3, no such evidence base exists at present. For a full list of which therapies fall into which Group please see Box 1 (Chapter 2).

III. Therapies in Group 1 are likely to respond to research as to effectiveness; indeed, some of them have already done so to a substantial degree and NHS provision is increasing for these disciplines. For some therapies in Group 2, NHS provision (especially in the care of the terminally ill) is already a reality. However, more work needs to be done to develop their regulatory structures and, in some cases, to encourage more research into their specific effects. For therapies in Group 3, the prospect of attracting research funding or NHS provision is likely to be difficult or, more probably, impossible (Chapters 3 and 7).

IV. The interests of the public in their use of CAM will be best served by improved regulatory structures for many of the professions concerned. Although there is evidence of progress across many fronts, the Committee found considerable diversity of standards, with an unacceptable fragmentation in some therapies, especially in Groups 2 and 3. In the best interests of their patients such therapies must each strive to unite under a single voluntary regulatory body with the features we highlight (Chapter 5).

V. In a few cases regulation by statute may be appropriate. Our main criteria for preferring such a route are first, the possible risk to the public from poor practice; second, a pre-existing robust voluntary regulatory system; and third, the presence of a credible evidence base. We consider that acupuncture and herbal medicine comply with these criteria and we support their moves towards statutory regulation. In time, such regulation may become appropriate for homeopathy (Chapter 5).

VI. We have learnt that the regulation of herbal products presents significant challenges for public health. In particular it is difficult for the public to identify remedies of adequate quality, or to distinguish those with medicines licences from those sold as foods or those currently exempt from licensing. We recommend that the Medicines Control Agency (MCA) help the public identify regulated products more clearly. We also recommend that the law against illegal or misleading labelling be rigorously enforced. We further support the MCA and the Government in their advocacy of a new draft directive in the European Union that would more effectively regulate this complex sector (Chapter 5).

VII. There are currently no clear guidelines relating to the regulation and training in CAM practice amongst statutory regulated health professionals (such as doctors and nurses) who wish to incorporate a CAM therapy into their personal clinical repertoire. We recommend that the existing regulatory bodies in each of the healthcare professions should develop clear guidelines on competence and training in the CAM disciplines and on the position they take in relation to their members' activities in CAM (Chapter 5).

VIII. Many CAM therapies are based on theories about their modes of action that are not congruent with current scientific knowledge. That is not to say that new scientific knowledge may not emerge in the future. Nevertheless as a Select Committee on Science and Technology we must make it clear from the outset that while we accept that some CAM therapies, notably osteopathy, chiropractic and herbal medicine, have established efficacy in the treatment of a limited range of ailments, we remain sceptical about the modes of action of most of the others. We therefore emphasise that in recommending the regulation of training in CAM we specifically exclude training in the asserted modes of action of many CAM therapies. We do so because regulation could lead to a misleading public perception of improved status; such regulation is in fact an attempt to safeguard the public.

IX. CAM training courses vary unacceptably in content, depth and duration. Only a concerted partnership between higher educational institutions and properly regulated professions as validating bodies will adequately ensure that any CAM practitioner is well trained. Accredited training of CAM practitioners is vital in ensuring that the public are protected from incompetent practitioners. We hope that the recommendations in Chapter 6 will help guide the CAM professional bodies in developing and supporting consistently good quality training programmes (Chapter 6).

X. Many of the CAM therapies and especially, in our view, those in Group 1 and some in Group 2, share common concerns such as a need to improve research awareness amongst practitioners, a need to understand the ethical aspects of healthcare and the nature of the therapeutic relationship. If each such therapy develops one professional regulatory body responsible for supervising all training in that discipline, as we recommend that they should, this should result in core competencies covering these topics being defined for each therapy. The extent of training required will depend on how far a therapy claims to be independent of medical supervision and diagnosis (Chapter 6).

XI. Conventional healthcare practitioners should become familiar with CAM therapies, their potential uses, and their main weaknesses and dangers. We consider that the provision of CAM familiarisation in schools of medicine and nursing is currently too uneven. We make recommendations to the regulatory bodies concerned to rectify this position. We also highlight the importance of Continuing Professional Development in order that existing healthcare professionals are aware of this area and can advise their patients accordingly (Chapter 6).

XII. Very little high-quality CAM research exists; reasons for this may include: a lack of training in the principles and methods of research; inadequate research funding and a poor research infrastructure within the CAM sector. Another contributing factor may be methodological issues, with many CAM practitioners believing that conventional research methods are not suitable tools with which to investigate CAM. In the light of these problems we recommend that a central mechanism for co-ordinating and advising on CAM research and for making available research training opportunities be established, with resourcing from the Government and, possibly, the charitable sector. Such a body could implement various means of aiding CAM research. Training CAM practitioners in methods and principles of appropriate research disciplines will undoubtedly increase research activity in this area as will attracting mainstream investigators into CAM research. This will only happen if sufficient funds are available and an appropriate academic infrastructure is established (Chapter 7).

XIII. CAM faces problems in attracting research funds from industry and charity. Many of our witnesses suggested that without dedicated funds for CAM research, the research infrastructure for CAM will remain poor. We have recommended that the NHS R&D directorate and the MRC should pump-prime this area with dedicated research funding to develop a few centres of excellence for conducting CAM research on appropriate disciplines. These centres of excellence could be based on the model pioneered in this area by the very successful National Center for Complementary and Alternative Medicine in the USA (Chapter 7).

XIV. We recommend that CAM should attempt to build up an evidence base with the same rigour as is required of conventional medicine, using both randomised controlled trials (RCTs) and other research designs which we discuss (see paras 7.10 – 7.30). We believe that those therapies in Group 1 are likely to command the highest proportion of research resources. Other therapies will need to build up their respective evidence bases with small preliminary studies before large scale studies are justifiable (Chapter 7).

XV. There is a clear need for more effective guidance for the public as to what does or does not work and what is or is not safe in CAM. There is no central information provision for patients and healthcare practitioners; thus the media and other unregulated sources have an undue influence on opinion in the field. We are not convinced that many CAM professions themselves are yet in the position to provide balanced and consensual views on these issues of public interest. The obvious place to turn to for such advice is the NHS and we believe that this responsibility has not yet been adequately fulfilled. We recommend that central resources be directed either through the Government or in partnership with a neutral body to ensure that the public has access to balanced and fair advice on CAM (Chapter 8).

XVI. One of the main dangers of CAM is that patients could miss out on conventional medical diagnosis and treatment because they choose only to consult a CAM practitioner. We recommend that all NHS provision of CAM should continue to be through GP referral (or referral from other healthcare professionals working in the NHS in primary, secondary or tertiary care) (Chapter 9).

XVII. We recommend that the CAM disciplines define their respective areas of competence and confirm their willingness to refer patients to conventional medical care when appropriate (Chapter 6).

XVIII. Another actual or potential risk arising from CAM use is that patients may not tell their GPs that they are receiving other treatment, and may thus risk complications from drug interactions. In the past, the tendency for conventional practitioners to be sceptical or even sometimes hostile to CAM may have contributed to the likelihood of patients being secretive about their use of CAM. We urge CAM practitioners and GPs to keep an open mind about each other's ability to help their patients and to exchange information about treatment programmes and their perceptions of the healthcare needs of patients (Chapter 9).

XIX. NHS provision of CAM is currently very patchy and has been in some cases adversely affected by the recent NHS reforms in Primary Care. We heard much evidence about how to recommend which therapies should be made available on the NHS. In formulating our recommendations on the issue of the availability of such therapies on the NHS by GP referral, or by referral from healthcare professionals in secondary or tertiary care, we concluded that in view of the variable evidence bases which at present exist it might initially be unfair to restrict NHS provision only to those with firmly established efficacy. We recommend, however, that only those CAM therapies which are statutory regulated or have robust mechanisms of voluntary self-regulation should be available through public funding (Chapter 9).

CHAPTER 1: INTRODUCTION

What is Complementary and Alternative Medicine?

1.1 Aspirin (acetylsalicylic acid) was the first synthetic chemical drug. It was manufactured by Bayer in Germany, patented and put on the market in 1899. Until then treatment in Western medicine, as in all other forms of medical practice, including Chinese and Ayurvedic medicine, was very largely based on the use of herbs supplemented by preparations of metals and occasionally animal preparations. The preparations in the Herbal of Dioscorides published in 55AD remained largely unchanged in Western pharmacopeias until the twentieth century. There was very considerable variation in the range of herbs available in Eastern countries and their pharmacopeias reflected this. But apart from such differences, the aims were the same, namely to use the herbs that were available for their effects in ameliorating the symptoms of disease.

1.2 In virtually all systems of medicine the claims made for the efficacy of such preparations in treating a wide range of diseases and symptoms usually lacked any clear supporting evidence or a sound foundation. This was reinforced by the tendency, still found in the Eastern systems of medicine today, to prescribe a mixture of many different herbs rather than a single remedy. Quinine (derived from cinchona bark) for malaria, digitalis (from the foxglove) for heart failure and opium (from the poppy) for pain relief were exceptions but even their efficacy was only established after many years of empirical use. Before the introduction of the National Health Service (NHS) in 1948, the provision of primary medical care in the United Kingdom was very uneven. Nevertheless, many doctors were able to find ample time to spend with their patients. They made many house visits and came to know much about the families for whom they cared, both medically and socially. Their principal method of caring for their patients, apart from using the range of herbal remedies available, was the provision of what has been referred to commonly as "tender loving care" (TLC) to aid natural recovery, namely to supplement the "vis medicatrix naturae"[1].

1.3 The rate of development in Western countries of new synthetic chemical drugs has increased steadily since the introduction of aspirin. Western medicine now has an armamentarium of remedies that provides the means of preventing or curing many specific diseases and also of mitigating the symptoms of many more. This has not happened to any major extent in any other systems of medicine, although new and effective herbal remedies are still being discovered and are becoming available to complement the enormous variety of effective synthetic drugs which are now being used in conventional Western medicine.

1.4 In parallel with the increased availability of synthetic drugs, there have been remarkable developments in surgery. These escalated following the development of effective anaesthesia, which made complex surgery possible for the first time. The range of feasible surgical interventions has increased dramatically and offers a new prospect of radical cures or mitigation of many maladies. There has also been a dramatic increase in knowledge of the biochemical or molecular origin of many diseases so that new diagnostic tests have emerged, many dependent upon measuring the concentration of various chemical entities in the blood stream, or upon the use of DNA recombinant technology.

1.5 There are however many common diseases, mostly chronic, for which new drugs and surgical interventions have so far failed to provide outcomes that are satisfactory for many patients. Among these are the various forms of arthritis, low back pain, asthma, some forms of cancer and many more.

1.6 Modern Western medicine is both complex and expensive. Increasing pressures on an under-doctored National Health Service (NHS) are now such that the average primary care physician has very little time to spend with each patient in consultation in order to offer the attention and 'tender loving care' which were important therapeutic weapons for his predecessors. When he or she diagnoses a serious or acute condition known to be amenable to modern treatment, the patient will usually be referred to an appropriate specialist, although some such problems can increasingly be handled effectively in primary care. When a chronic complaint is diagnosed it is often treated symptomatically with a prescription drug. Furthermore in a group practice patients may sometimes see different doctors on each occasion they attend, and thus lack a close therapeutic relationship with a single doctor. Added to this is the fact that many conventional medical and surgical interventions, as well as effective synthetic drugs, and even some of herbal origin, produce in some patients troublesome and distressing side-effects which may occasionally even have fatal consequences. Such adverse reactions are usually less common with complementary and alternative therapies. The benefit-risk ratio must be taken into account.

---

[1]   The body's natural healing power.

1.7 It is not, therefore, surprising that the satisfaction expressed by many patients with conventional medicine is often not as good as it was in the past. It is probable that this is one of the principal reasons why there has been such a marked increase in the numbers of people who turn to other systems of medicine or to complementary or alternative medicine to replace or supplement their conventional medical advice. It is these complementary and alternative disciplines that we examine in this report.

1.8 Complementary and Alternative Medicine (CAM) is a title used to refer to a diverse group of health-related therapies and disciplines which are not considered to be a part of mainstream medical care. Other terms sometimes used to describe them include 'natural medicine', 'non-conventional medicine' and 'holistic medicine'. However, CAM is currently the term used most often, and hence we have adopted it on our Report. CAM embraces those therapies that may either be provided alongside conventional medicine (complementary) or which may, in the view of their practitioners, act as a substitute for it. Alternative disciplines purport to provide diagnostic information as well as offering therapy.

1.9 This Inquiry was mounted because there is a widespread perception that CAM use is increasing not only in the United Kingdom but across the developed world. This appeared to raise several important questions of substantial significance in relation to public health policy.

1.10 Before assessing how CAM use could, or should, influence public health policy, a more quantitative picture of use in this area would be desirable. However, quantitative survey data in this area are somewhat patchy and are beset by questions of definition which are hard to resolve.

1.11 Several professional bodies have attempted to define CAM. The British Medical Association (BMA) report *Complementary Medicine: New Approaches to Good Practice* suggests that although the term 'complementary therapies' is familiar to the public, a more accurate term might be 'non-conventional therapies'. The BMA defines these as: "those forms of treatment which are not widely used by the conventional healthcare professions, and the skills of which are not taught as part of the undergraduate curriculum of conventional medical and paramedical healthcare courses"[2]. This definition is now unsatisfactory as the use of some of the therapies traditionally considered to be non-conventional is growing amongst doctors (although practice varies widely). Some medical schools are now offering CAM familiarisation courses to undergraduate medical students while some also offer modules specifically on CAM.

1.12 Professor Edzard Ernst, who holds a Chair in CAM at Exeter University, provided the following definition: "Complementary medicine is diagnosis, treatment and/or prevention which complements mainstream medicine by contributing to a common whole, by satisfying a demand not met by orthodoxy or by diversifying the conceptual frameworks of medicine"[3]. This definition helps to elucidate the aims of complementary medicine, but it does not cover alternative therapies which do not seek to contribute to a common whole but which are offered by their practitioners as an alternative to conventional medicine. A more encompassing definition of CAM is provided by the Cochrane Collaboration as: "a broad domain of healing resources that encompasses all health systems, modalities, and practices and their accompanying theories and beliefs, other than those intrinsic to the politically dominant health systems of a particular society or culture in a given historical period".

1.13 The CAM community has been struggling for fifteen years to come up with a single definition of CAM agreed by all, but with no success. Therefore, when setting up this Inquiry we decided not to begin with a precise definition of CAM. Instead we began with a list of therapies which we thought were commonly considered to fall within the field of CAM and issued this list with our Call for Evidence (see Box 1). Additional disciplines have subsequently been added in the light of evidence received (identified by an asterisk in Box 1). In making the list of therapies we have provisionally grouped the ones we regard principally as complementary separately from the ones we regard principally as alternative. While no firm distinction is possible, we regard the complementary disciplines as those which usually, if not invariably, complement conventional medical treatment, while the alternative disciplines are those which purport to offer diagnostic and therapeutic alternatives to conventional medicine.

Growing Use of CAM in the United Kingdom

1.14 We have heard much evidence to the effect that we are now experiencing a rapid increase in the use of CAM across the Western World. There are limited data on the exact levels of use and much

---

[2] British Medical Association *Complementary Medicine: New Approaches to Good Practice* (Oxford University Press, 1993).

[3] Ernst, E. et al. 'Complementary Medicine – A Definition' [letter] in *The British Journal of General Practice* (1995; 5:506).

of the information that is available does not refer to the United Kingdom. However, some surveys have been conducted and are reviewed briefly below, in an attempt to achieve a snapshot of existing CAM use. This has helped to inform subsequent conclusions about the implications this evidence may have in relation to future healthcare policy.

1.15 Caution should be exercised when making comparisons. The results of the different surveys reveal a wide range in the extent of CAM use. This may partly be due to different definitions of CAM being used, different methods being used to implement the survey, the population surveyed and the range of therapies considered. We have therefore provided a brief summary of the specific CAM disciplines being considered by each survey at the beginning of each review. It must also be noted that these surveys take no account of the increasing use by the public of self-medication through the purchase of conventional over-the-counter remedies such as analgesics, cough medicines, antacids and vitamins. We have not attempted to compare in detail the extent of such self-medication with the extent of CAM self-medication. However, the Royal Pharmaceutical Society tell us that in 1999 £2318 million was spent on non-prescription medicine. They also told us that the non-prescription market has made increasing profits over the past four years for which they had figures.

BRITISH SURVEYS

1.16 In 1999 Mr Simon Mills[4] and Ms Sarah Budd at the Centre for Complementary Health Studies at Exeter University were commissioned by the Department of Health to conduct a study of the professional organisation of CAM bodies in the United Kingdom[5]. This was a follow-up to a study conducted on the same subject three years earlier[6]. It looked at how many people were working as CAM practitioners. Its results suggest that there are approximately 50,000 CAM practitioners in the United Kingdom, that there are approximately 10,000 statutory registered health professionals who practise some form of CAM in the United Kingdom and that up to 5 million patients have consulted a CAM practitioner in the last year. Hence there are two considerations to consider: the number of practitioners and the number of patients. Patients can access CAM either through professional CAM practitioners, through other health professionals (e.g. doctors, nurses and physiotherapists who offer CAM services) or through the purchase of over-the-counter preparations.

1.17 A telephone survey of 1204 randomly selected British adults was conducted for the BBC in 1999[7]. This survey did not specify which therapies it classed as CAM; instead respondents were asked if they had used 'alternative or complementary medicines or therapies' within the last year. This was followed by an open-ended question asking: 'What specifically do you or have you used or done?' Therefore the definition of CAM was left up to the respondent. This survey's results are summarised in Table 1.

Table 1: Use of CAM in the United Kingdom

	1999 (%)
Use of any CAM in past 12 months	20
Of which: *	
Herbal medicine	34
Aromatherapy	21
Homeopathy	17
Acupuncture / acupressure	14
Massage	6
Reflexology	6
Osteopathy	4
Chiropractic	3

Source: nationally representative random telephone survey of 1204 British adults, commissioned by the BBC.

* Percentages of those who had used CAM. It must be noted that some individuals use more than one therapy and thus the numbers above do not add up to 100.

---

4   Simon Mills, Director of the Centre for Complementary Health Studies at Exeter University, was one of the specialist advisers to the Sub-Committee who prepared this report.

5   Mills, S. & Peacock, W. *Professional Organisation of Complementary and Alternative Medicine in the UK 1997: A Report to the Department of Health* (University of Exeter, 1997).

6   Budd, S. & Mills, S. *Professional Organisation of Complementary and Alternative Medicine in the United Kingdom 2000: A Second Report to the Department of Health* (University of Exeter, 2000).

7   Ernst, E. & White, A. 'The BBC Survey of Complementary Medicine Use in the UK' in *Complementary Therapies in Medicine*, 8 (2000), 32-36.

1.18 However, this survey did not expand on whether the treatment was accessed through the purchase of over-the-counter remedies or through a professional consultation. This survey also found that the average amount of money each CAM user spent on CAM was approximately £14 per month with a large proportion of users (37%) spending less than five pounds per month. The authors extrapolated this information to the whole nation and estimated that the United Kingdom has an annual expenditure of £1.6 billion on CAM.

1.19 Another survey[8] of CAM use in England (not the United Kingdom) used a questionnaire sent out as a postal survey to 5010 randomly selected adults and received 2668 usable responses (a corrected response rate of 53%). This survey asked respondents whether they had visited a practitioner of one of eight named therapies in the last twelve months. The named therapies were acupuncture, chiropractic, homeopathy, medical herbalism, hypnotherapy, osteopathy, aromatherapy and reflexology. The survey also asked for information on whether respondents had purchased any over-the-counter, herbal, or homeopathic remedies. Results showed that 13.6% of respondents had visited a practitioner of one of the eight named therapies in the preceding 12 months, and overall 28.3% of respondents had either visited a CAM therapist or had purchased an over-the-counter remedy. The most commonly consulted CAM therapists were osteopaths (4.3% of respondents), chiropractors (3.6%), aromatherapists (3.5%), reflexologists (2.4%), and acupuncturists (1.6%). Of the respondents, 8.6% had bought an over-the-counter homeopathic remedy and 19.8% had bought an over-the-counter herbal remedy. The NHS paid for an estimated 10% of the visits to practitioners but the authors estimate that £450 million worth of out-of-pocket expenditure was used on six of the principal therapies (excluding aromatherapy and reflexology) during the preceding year.

1.20 In their evidence to us the Royal Pharmaceutical Society discussed a report from 1999 on over-the-counter sale of CAM preparations prepared for industry by Mintel Marketing Intelligence (Q 1313). This report found that retail sales of complementary medicine (herbals, homeopathic preparations and aromatherapy essential oils) totalled £93m in 1998. A breakdown of this figure showed that £50m had come from sales of herbal medicines, £23m from homeopathic medicines and £20m from aromatherapy essential oils. The report also showed that these figures were increasing and that the total revenue was up 50% from £63m in 1994. Overall retail sales in 2000 were predicted to reach £109m and predictions for 2002 were £126m[9].

1.21 These rather limited data seem to support the idea that CAM use in the United Kingdom is high and is increasing. This conclusion is supported by anecdotal evidence received from many of our witnesses including the Foundation for Integrated Medicine (FIM),[10] the NHS Alliance and the Department of Health, confirming that the public are very interested in this area. A glance at any women's magazine will reveal pages of information dealing with dietary supplements and alternative medicine clinics. However, as mentioned earlier, a more authoritative picture is desirable. Apart from the data discussed above there is little other evidence available about usage of CAM in the United Kingdom and a comparison with the extent of usage of self-medication with conventional over-the-counter remedies would be useful. **More detailed quantitative information is required on the levels of CAM use in the United Kingdom, in order to inform the public and healthcare policy-makers and we recommend that suitable national studies be commissioned to obtain this information.** Information from other developed countries is also relevant.

UNITED STATES SURVEYS

1.22 In the United States Eisenberg, David and Ettner[11] conducted two national telephone surveys of two randomly selected sets of adults, surveying levels of CAM usage in 1990 and 1997 respectively. They questioned respondents on their use of sixteen 'alternative therapies' and defined accessing alternative medicine as having used at least one of the sixteen therapies (either as an over-

---

[8]   Thomas, K.J., Nicholl, J.P. & Coleman, P. 'Use of and Expenditure on Complementary Medicine in England – A Population-Based Survey'. *Complementary Therapies in Medicine* (In Press).

[9]   The fastest growing sales figures were for essential oils, which had almost doubled in sales volume in real terms since 1993. Sales of homeopathic products had grown at a steady rate of around 4% per annum and those of herbal medicines were growing at a steady rate of about 10% per annum.

[10] The Foundation for Integrated Medicine was formed at the personal initiative of HRH The Prince of Wales, who is now its President. The aim of the Foundation for Integrated Medicine is to promote the development and integrated delivery of safe, effective and efficient forms of healthcare to patients and their families through encouraging greater collaboration between all forms of healthcare. The Foundation operates as a forum, actively promoting and supporting discussion, and as a centre to facilitate development and action. Its objective is to "enable individuals to promote, restore and maintain health and well-being through integrating the approaches of orthodox, complementary and alternative therapies".

[11] Eisenberg, D.M., Davis, R.B., Ettner, S.L. et al. 'Trends in Alternative Medicine Use in the United States, 1990-1997: Results of a Follow-up National Survey' in *The Journal of the American Medical Association*, 280 (1998) 1569-1575.

the-counter preparation or through a professional consultation) within the previous year. The sixteen therapies included several that we did not include in our Call for Evidence, e.g. mega-vitamins, self-help groups, imagery, and commercial and lifestyle diets. Their remit did not include osteopathy which was included in our Call for Evidence, and which is generally regarded as a mainstream medical speciality in the USA.

1.23 The results of this survey are shown in Table 2. In both the 1990 and the 1997 surveys, alternative therapies were used mainly for chronic conditions such as back pain, allergies, anxiety, depression and headaches. The authors of the survey found that extrapolation of their results to the entire population of the USA suggested a 47.3% total increase in visits to alternative practitioners, from 427 million to 629 million (which was more than the number of visits to all US primary care physicians). Out-of-pocket expenditure on alternative therapies was estimated at $27.0 billion in 1997.

Table 2: Use of CAM in the USA

	1990 (%)	1997 (%)
Use of any CAM in past 12 months of which[‡]	33.8[†]	42.1[†]
Relaxation techniques	13.1	16.3
Herbal medicine	2.5	12.1
Massage	6.9	11.1
Chiropractic	10.1	11.0
Spiritual healing	4.2	7.0
Homeopathy	0.7	3.4
Acupuncture	0.4	1.0

Source: two nationally representative random household telephone surveys.

[†] *Percentages of the total sample population (1539 for the 1990 data; 2055 in 1997).*

[‡] *Table shows selected figures relating to the top five therapies based on the 1997 survey, plus (for comparison with United Kingdom statistics) figures for homeopathy and acupuncture.*

Reasons for Accessing CAM

SURVEY DATA

1.24 A national postal survey of 1035 adults which was designed specifically to find out why patients use CAM was conducted in the USA in 1998[12]. The survey asked about respondents' need for control over their own health; their philosophical orientation towards religion, spirituality, mind and body; their belief in the efficacy of conventional medicine and their general health and demographic statistics. A multiple regression analysis was then used to identify predictors of alternative healthcare use. The most significant predictor was higher educational status, followed by overall health status. Chronic health problems such as anxiety, back problems, urinary tract problems and chronic pain were each also significant predictors of CAM use. Apart from health and social status the only other three significant predictors of CAM use were: being 'culturally creative'; having a holistic philosophical approach to life; and having had a 'transformational experience'. The author takes the view that dissatisfaction with conventional care was not the major factor leading to the use of CAM. He suggests that as well as being better educated and in poorer health, most users of CAM access these therapies because they find them to be 'more congruent with their own values, beliefs and philosophical orientations towards health and life'. However, it is worth noting that Astin never asked the critical question: " Has conventional medicine worked for you?" in his survey, even though he was assessing why people turned to CAM. The cost of conventional medical treatment in the USA may also have been another factor.

1.25 The BBC survey of CAM use in the United Kingdom also asked respondents who had used CAM what their main reason was for accessing CAM medicines or therapies[13]. Results are shown in Table 3.

---

[12] Astin, J.A. 'Why Patients use Alternative Medicine. Results of a National Survey'. *The Journal of the American Medical Association*, 279 (1998) 1548-1553.

[13] Ernst, E. & White, A. (2000) (*Op.cit.*).

Table 3 : Reasons for Using CAM

Reason	Percentage of those who use CAM
Helps or relieves injury / condition	25
Just like it	21
Find it relaxing	19
Good health / well-being generally	14
Preventative measure	12
Do not believe conventional medicine works	11
Doctor's recommendations / referral	11
To find out about other ways of life / new things	11
Way of life / part of lifestyle	8
Cannot get treatment on NHS / under conventional medicine	7

Source: nationally representative random telephone survey of 1204 British adults, commissioned by the BBC.

OTHER POSSIBLE EXPLANATIONS

1.26 Some evidence we have received has suggested reasons for CAM use that are neither to do with patient satisfaction with CAM, nor dissatisfaction with conventional medicine. Dr Thurstan Brewin (P 244) suggested that the current popularity of CAM is dictated by fashion, as is evidenced by the many articles and advertisements in the lay press. He also suggested that another reason for the rising trend in CAM utilisation relates to a cultural change with a renewed interest in the paranormal (e.g. astrology) which remains popular no matter how much evidence refutes it. He postulated that another factor in CAM's popularity is the increased anxiety about health across society, despite the longer and safer lives which people now lead. He therefore suggested that much of CAM's popularity lies with the 'worried well', a suggestion others have also made.

1.27 In their oral evidence to us the General Medical Council (GMC) put forward that one other reason for CAM's popularity may be the general attitude of society towards science (Q 1036). They suggested that in some areas of society there is a flight from science, fuelled by unbalanced and inaccurate articles in the media and by the unsubstantiated claims from some environmental groups. The subject of society's flight from science was tackled by this Committee last year and is discussed in our previous report *Science and Society*[14].

1.28 It would be useful to have more research on why the public are increasingly using CAM in their healthcare regimes. At the moment the reasons are unclear, but the answer to this question is important as it may have implications for the NHS, conventional healthcare practitioners and CAM practitioners, who wish to meet their patients' needs more comprehensively.

Approach of This Report

1.29 This report does not consider the clinical efficacy of particular products or therapies except insofar as evidence is available to inform policy. We shall return to our reasons for this later in the report.

1.30 Whatever the reasons behind the popularity of CAM it is clear that there is an increasing number of patients and practitioners who are each involved in this area of healthcare. It is this high level of public interest that has prompted our Inquiry, raising important public policy questions that we have been charged with considering:

(i) In an age where conventional medical research is advancing rapidly with major benefits for patient care and increasing life expectancy, why are people using CAM and for what are they using it?

(ii) Since most statutory controls pertain to conventional medical and other healthcare practitioners and their relevant organisations, are current regulations adequate to provide a safe service for patients using CAM?

(iii) Does current medical training prepare doctors, nurses and others to answer patients' questions about CAM? Do they have enough information? Should their training include familiarisation with CAM?

---

[14] See our Report: *Science & Society*, 3rd Report 1999-2000, HL Paper 38.

(iv)   How well developed is the training of CAM practitioners? Are appropriate structures in place to support high-quality training? Are proper codes of practice being developed? Are appropriate accreditation processes in place to protect the patient? Are issues of Continued Professional Development being considered?

(v)   Is the state of CAM research adequate? Is appropriate research being carried out to investigate efficacy and to ensure that patients are receiving safe, effective treatments? Are current research methods appropriate for CAM research? Is research funding available and is the research infrastructure there to support work in this area?

(vi)   Should CAM's popularity among the public result in an increase in NHS CAM provision? If so, how should CAM be delivered? Should it invariably be complementary, perhaps by reference to CAM practitioners by doctors in primary care, or is there any case for the provision of alternative medicine on the NHS? Will NHS reforms change how CAM is provided on the NHS?

Conduct of this Inquiry

1.31 This report was prepared by Sub-Committee I, whose members are listed in Appendix 7, with their declarations of interest. We received evidence from a wide range of individuals and organisations, to all of whom we are grateful; they are listed in Appendix 8. The written evidence received up until 1st February 2000 is printed in HL Paper 48. The oral evidence received at 21 public hearings, and the written evidence received after 1st February is published in HL Paper 118.

1.32 We record our gratitude to our specialist advisers: Professor Stephen Holgate, MRC Professor of Immunopharmacology, University of Southampton and a member of the Board of the Foundation for Integrated Medicine; and Mr Simon Mills, Director of the Centre for Complementary Health Studies, University of Exeter, and a member of the Council of the Foundation for Integrated Medicine. We also wish to express particular gratitude to those who met us at the University of Exeter, the University of Southampton, the Centre for Complementary Health Studies at Southampton, the Marylebone Health Centre, London, and the Glasgow Homeopathic Hospital.

CHAPTER 2: DISCIPLINES EXAMINED

Definitions of the Various CAM Therapies

2.1 The therapeutic disciplines which were either included in the Committee's Call for Evidence or from whom evidence was received are listed in Box 1. The list is not intended to be all-inclusive but rather it is an attempt to provide an indication and framework of the main types of therapy we have considered without attempting to resolve the difficulties inherent in formulating an exact definition of CAM. We broadly follow the definitions of each therapy given in Box 1. The Committee was happy to receive evidence from representatives of any therapy or discipline that considered itself to be either complementary or alternative to mainstream medicine. Broadly, in the opinion of the Committee, these therapies and disciplines fall into three broad groups:

- *The first group* embraces what may be called the principal disciplines, two of which, osteopathy and chiropractic, are already regulated in their professional activity and education by Acts of Parliament. The others are acupuncture, herbal medicine and homeopathy. Our evidence has indicated that each of these therapies claim to have an individual diagnostic approach and that these therapies are seen as the 'Big 5' by most of the CAM world.

- *The second group* contains therapies which are most often used to complement conventional medicine and do not purport to embrace diagnostic skills. It includes aromatherapy; the Alexander Technique; body work therapies, including massage; counselling; stress therapy; hypnotherapy; reflexology and probably shiatsu; meditation and healing.

- *The third group* embraces those other disciplines in Box 1 which purport to offer diagnostic information as well as treatment and which, in general, favour a philosophical approach and are indifferent to the scientific principles of conventional medicine, and through which various and disparate frameworks of disease causation and its management are proposed. These therapies can be split into two sub-groups. Group 3a includes long-established and traditional systems of healthcare such as Ayurvedic medicine and Traditional Chinese medicine. Group 3b covers other alternative disciplines which lack any credible evidence base such as crystal therapy, iridology, radionics, dowsing and kinesiology.

2.2 We will be using these groups as our basis for the discussion of the different therapies throughout this report.

2.3 The evidence that we received from almost all the different therapies said that at the point of diagnosis, if the practitioners thought that their treatment would not work, they would refer their patients to an orthodox medical practitioner. We were encouraged by this sentiment, even though it was not universal.

Box 1

Short and Simplified Descriptions of CAM Disciplines

Group 1: Professionally Organised Alternative Therapies

Acupuncture — Originating from China, acupuncture involves inserting small needles into various points in the body to stimulate nerve impulses. Traditional Chinese acupuncture is based on the idea of 'qi' (vital energy) which is said to travel around the body along 'meridians' which the acupuncture points affect. Western Acupuncture uses the same needling technique but is based on affecting nerve impulses and the central nervous system; acupuncture may be used in the West as an anaesthetic-agent and also as an analgesic.

Chiropractic — Used almost entirely to treat musculo-skeletal complaints through adjusting muscles, tendons and joints and using manipulation and massage techniques. Diagnostic procedures include case histories, conventional clinical examination and x-rays. Chiropractic was originally based on the idea that 'reduced nerve flow' led to disease.

Herbal medicine — A system of medicine which uses various remedies derived from plants and plant extracts to treat disorders and maintain good health. Another term for this type of treatment is phytotherapy.

Homeopathy — A therapy based on the theory of treating like with like. Homeopathic remedies use highly diluted substances that if given in higher doses to a healthy person would produce the symptoms that the dilutions are being given to treat. In assessing the patient homeopaths often take into account a range of physical, emotional and lifestyle factors which contribute to the diagnosis.

Osteopathy — A system of diagnosis and treatment, usually by manipulation, that mainly focuses on musculo-skeletal problems, but a few schools claim benefits across a wider spectrum of disorders. Historically differs from chiropractic in its underlying theory that it is impairment of blood supply and not nerve supply that leads to problems. However in practice there is less difference than might be assumed. Mainstream osteopathy focuses on musculo-skeletal problems; but prior to osteopathy gaining statutory protection of title, other branches of this therapy purported to diagnose and treat a range of disorders. One such branch is now known as cranio-sacral therapy, which should be considered as a distinct therapy which would fall into Group 3.

Box 1 continued

Group 2: Complementary Therapies

Alexander Technique — Based on a theory that the way a person uses their body affects their general health. This technique encourages people to optimise their health by teaching them to stand, sit and move according to the body's 'natural design and function'. This is, in essence, a taught technique, rather than a therapy.

Aromatherapy — Use of plant extract essential oils inhaled, used as a massage oil, or occasionally ingested. Common in France but practised there by medical doctors only. Can be used to alleviate specific symptoms or as a relaxant.

Bach and other flower remedies —— The theory behind flower remedies is that flowers contain the life force of the plant and this is imprinted into water through sun infusion which is used to make the flower remedy. Flower remedies are often used to help patients let go of negative thoughts; usually flower remedies are ingested.

Body work therapies, including massage — Therapies that use rubbing, kneading and the application of pressure to address aches, pains and musculo-skeletal problems. Often used as a relaxant.

Counselling stress therapy — A series of psychical therapies that attempt to help patients to work through their thoughts and to reflect on their lives so as to maximise wellbeing.

Hypnotherapy — The use of hypnosis in treating behavioural disease and dysfunction, principally mental disorders.

Meditation — A series of techniques used to relax a patient to facilitate deep reflection and a clearing of the mind (see Maharishi Ayurvedic Medicine below).

Reflexology — A system of massage of the feet based on the idea that there are invisible zones running vertically through the body, so that each organ has a corresponding location in the foot. It has also been claimed to stimulate blood supply and relieve tension.

Shiatsu — A type of massage originating from Japan which aims to stimulate the body's healing ability by applying light pressure to points across the body. Relies on the meridian system of 'qi' in a similar way to traditional Chinese medicine and acupuncture.

Healing — A system of spiritual healing, sometimes based on prayer and religious beliefs, that attempts to tackle illness through non-physical means, usually by directing thoughts towards an individual. Often involves 'the laying on of hands'.

Maharishi Ayurvedic Medicine * — A system which promotes transcendental meditation, derived from the Vedic tradition in India. Recommends the use of herbal preparations similar to those used in Ayurvedic Medicine (see below) and Traditional Chinese medicine (see below).

Nutritional medicine — Term used to cover the use of nutritional methods to address and prevent disease. Uses diets and nutritional supplements. Often used to address allergies and chronic digestive problems. The difference between nutritional medicine and dietetics is that nutritional therapists work independently in accordance with naturopathic principles and focus on disorders which they believe can be attributed to nutritional deficiency, food intolerance or toxic overload. They believe these three factors are involved in a wide range of health problems. Dieticians usually work under medical supervision, using diets to encourage healthy eating and tackle a narrower range of diseases. Nutritional therapists often use exclusion diets and herbal remedies to tackle patients' problems.

Yoga — A system of adopting postures with related exercises designed to promote spiritual and physical well-being.

Box 1 continued

Group 3: Alternative Disciplines

3a: *Long-established and traditional systems of healthcare*

Anthroposophical medicine — 'Anthroposophy' describes people in terms of their physicality, their soul and their spirit. Anthroposophical medicine aims to stimulate a person's natural healing forces through studying the influence of their soul and spirit on their physical body.

Ayurvedic Medicine — An ancient discipline, originating in India, based upon the principle of mind-spirit-body interaction and employing natural herbs, usually mixtures, in treatment.

*Chinese Herbal Medicine** — (See Traditional Chinese medicine below) A tradition of medicine used for thousands of years in China, which has its own system of diagnosis. Uses combinations of herbs to address a wide range of health problems.

Eastern Medicine (Tibb)* — Tibb is a tradition which synthesises elements of health philosophy from Egypt, India, China and classical Greece. It literally means 'nature'. The concept of wholeness and balance permeates the principle of Tibb. Imbalance is thought to cause disease. It is thought to occur on four levels: physical, emotional, mental and spiritual. Tibb uses a range of treatments including massage, manipulation, dietary advice and herbal medicine, and a psychotherapeutic approach to restore imbalances which are considered the cause of disease.

Naturopathy — A method of treatment based on the principle that the natural laws of life apply inside the body as well as outside. Uses a range of natural approaches including diet and herbs and encourages exposure to sun and fresh air to maximise the body's natural responses.

Traditional Chinese medicine — The theory behind Traditional Chinese medicine is that the body is a dynamic energy system. There are two types of energy – Yin qi and Yang qi - and it is thought if there is an imbalance in Yin and Yang qi then symptoms occur. Traditional Chinese medicine uses a number of treatment methods to restore the balance of Yin and Yang qi; these include acupuncture, herbal medicine, massage and the exercise technique Qigong.

3b: *Other alternative disciplines*

Crystal therapy — Based on the idea that crystals can absorb and transmit energy and that the body has a continuing fluctuating energy which the crystal helps to tune. Crystals are often placed in patterns around the patient's body to produce an energy network to adjust the patient's energy field or 'aura'.

Dowsing —— Traditionally used as a way to identify water sources underground. Is not itself a therapy but is used by a range of other disciplines to answer questions through intuitive skills. Often used in conjunction with Radionics.

Iridology — A method of diagnosing problems and assessing health status that relies on studying the iris of the eye and noting marks and changes.

Kinesiology — A manipulative therapy by which a patient's physical, chemical, emotional and nutritional imbalances are assessed by a system of muscle testing. The measurement of variation in stress resistance of groups of muscles is said to identify deficiencies and imbalances, thus enabling diagnosis and treatments by techniques which usually involve strengthening the body's energy through acupressure points.

Radionics — A type of instrument-assisted healing which attempts to detect disease before it has physically manifested itself. It is based on the belief that everyone is surrounded by an invisible energy field which the practitioner tunes into and then attempts to correct problems which have been identified. Practitioners believe it can be done over long distances. Instruments are a focus of the healer's intent and include sugar tablets which carry the healing 'idea'.

* We received evidence about these therapies although they were not included in our original Call for Evidence

2.4 An important point that has been raised in many submissions to us is that the list of therapies supplied in our Call for Evidence vary hugely in the amount and type of supportive evidence that is available (e.g. the Natural Medicines Society – P 155, and the British Medical Acupuncture Society – P 40). Many submissions assert that several of the disciplines, especially those listed in our third group, have no significant evidence base to support their claims for safety and efficacy and as such should not be considered alongside well-established and generally accepted CAM therapies such as osteopathy or chiropractic. Some submissions have complained that we have grouped all these therapies together and that many have nothing in common. They complain that it may be damaging to the better-established CAM professions and disciplines to group them with those which have no evidence base. We understand these views and it is for this reason that we propose the grouping given above.

2.5 It is well recognised by all of those involved in medical practice that many illnesses and diseases are self-limiting and are cured or have their worst effects overcome by the human body's natural resources (the vis medicatrix naturae) without specific medical intervention. In many others spontaneous remissions, often unexpected or even inexplicable, occur. When such events, however, follow the administration of various medicines or therapies, these developments are often used by practitioners of both conventional and CAM to suggest efficacy. But the history of medical science demonstrates clearly that anecdotal "evidence" of this nature is unsafe, even though there have been some cases in which such findings have led to well-designed research projects which have either confirmed or refuted the original anecdotal conclusion. Such research (appropriate methods are discussed in Chapter 7) is essential in order to produce a sound evidence base relating to efficacy.

2.6 Many CAM therapies are based on theories about their modes of action that are not congruent with current scientific knowledge. That is not to say that new scientific knowledge may not emerge in the future. Nevertheless as a Select Committee on Science and Technology we must make it clear from the outset that whilst we accept that some CAM therapies, notably osteopathy, chiropractic and herbal medicine, have scientifically established efficacy in the treatment of a limited number of ailments, we remain sceptical about the modes of action about many of the others.

2.7 While in the time available for our Inquiry we have not been able to carry out detailed investigations into all of the therapies listed in Box 1, and while the question of efficacy was not included in our initial terms of reference, in the absence of a credible evidence base it is our opinion that the therapies listed in our Group 3 cannot be supported unless and until convincing research evidence of efficacy based upon the results of well designed trials can be produced. Such evidence must be capable of showing that the effects of any therapeutic discipline are superior to those of the placebo effect (see paras 3.19-3.34). It is our view that for those therapies in our Group 3, no such evidence exists at present.

2.8 We are, however, satisfied that many therapies listed in our Group 2 give help and comfort to many patients when used in a complementary sense to support conventional medical care even though most of them also lack a firm scientific basis. Nevertheless in relieving stress, in alleviating side effects (for example of various forms of anti-cancer therapy) and in giving succour to the elderly and in palliative care they often fulfil an important role.

2.9 We recognise that deciding which therapeutic disciplines fall under the title of CAM is controversial. Those listed in our Call for Evidence ranged from several which are already being integrated into conventional medicine to others which are plainly far removed from conventional medicine, or even purport to offer an alternative system of healthcare. But we listed them together to reflect the fact that each was considered as a healthcare intervention not commonly considered to fall within the ambit of conventional medical practitioners. Most share common problems such as lack of research activity; a limited or non-existent evidence base; lack of acceptance by the conventional medical world; and sparse, if any, provision under the NHS. All experience these problems to different degrees.

2.10 We received a huge amount of written evidence from a wide range of interest groups, and we extended our deadline twice to give as many people as possible the opportunity to submit evidence. Over 55 oral hearings were held. The issues considered in this report are intended to be relevant to any therapeutic discipline which aims to improve the health of individuals or populations and which is not traditionally considered part of conventional medicine.

2.11 This report discusses not only therapies that are complementary or alternative to conventional medicine; we also took evidence from people who used CAM in dental and veterinary practice.

Differing Philosophies

2.12 CAM therapies may differ from conventional medicine not only in their methods but also in some of their underlying philosophies. The way that many CAM disciplines define health, illness and the healing process can depart significantly from the beliefs that underlie the practice of conventional medicine. It is essential to consider the different paradigms from which conventional medicine and CAM approach healthcare as these have implications for research and integration. A spectrum exists between reductionism and holism and different practices in both conventional medicine and CAM span the spectrum.

2.13 We are aware that it is a fallacy to say that there is one philosophy that underlies all CAM disciplines. Evidence submitted to us by Mr Roger Newman Turner, a practising osteopath and naturopath, suggests that the term "complementary and alternative medicine" defines the therapies by their position outside of conventional medicine, rather than by any common philosophy. In fact, the CAM therapies come from hugely diverse backgrounds. However, there are some principles which most CAM therapies seem to share (P 87).

2.14 The World Health Organisation's definition of health is: "a state of complete physical, mental and social well-being, and not merely the absence of disease or infirmity"[15]. However, Mr Newman Turner pointed out that conventional medical treatment has focused on the elimination of symptoms and disease processes. Many CAM therapies emphasise the other features of the definition of "health" with attributes such as good energy, happiness and a sense of wellbeing being more central outcomes. Moreover the emphasis of much of CAM is often on strengthening the whole organism rather than directly attacking the pathology (such as an infection or tumour). CAM therapies use different vocabularies to understand these emphases, with treatment concepts such as detoxification and tonification, and with different cultural concepts of "energy" as recuperative forces in the body (notably in forms of medicine originating in Asia).

2.15 Most CAM therapies also apply a non-Cartesian view of health, making less distinction between the body, mind and spirit as distinct sources of disease. The language used in CAM often tends to imply that all these dimensions of the human condition should be viewed in the same therapeutic frame. Evidence we have received from other witnesses has also stressed repeatedly that CAM therapies take a highly individualistic approach to treatment. This often results in patients receiving a combination of treatments tailored to their specific needs. This is different from the conventional medical approach which may involve prescribing a standard drug and a similar treatment regime for patients with the same underlying pathology.

2.16 Nevertheless, many witnesses and organisations from conventional medicine emphasised the view that 'holistic medicine' is nothing more than good medical practice, and that conventional preventative medicine also concentrates on maintaining health and preventing disease. It is true that constraints of time, as we have mentioned, tend to reduce the attention that can be paid to the patients' emotional and social problems.

2.17 Some CAM therapies, and especially those in the Group 3a, have very specific philosophies that have evolved over centuries of use. Often these have developed into views about how the body functions and how disease is caused. Sometimes these are linked to the dominant religious philosophies of their country of origin. Examples include Ayurvedic medicine, and Traditional Chinese medicine. However, there is no established evidence base supporting these. The lack of an evidence base is even more evident in the case of those therapies we classify in Group 3b, and these must be subject to rigorous appraisal. Many conventional medical scientists, while accepting the validity of accumulative empirical observation, believe that those therapeutic disciplines that are based principally on abstract philosophy and not on scientific reasoning and experiment have little place in medicine. Professor Lewis Wolpert of the Academy of Medical Sciences told us that: "Medicine aims to base itself upon science. I am sorry that any complementary or alternative medicine procedure for which one can see no reasonable scientific basis should be supported" (Q 1404).

2.18 Evidence that we have received has suggested that conventional medicine allows any therapy proven to be effective to be subsumed into the medical curriculum (P 244). It is suggested that efficacious therapies are readily accepted and are not required to fit into any particular philosophy. Those who support the application of "normal science" pragmatism to CAM treatment have been accused by some complementary practitioners of trying to subsume the best of CAM therapy into their own paradigm, and yet of leaving much of what CAM sees as important (its philosophy) out in the cold.

---

[15] www.who.int/aboutwho/en/definition.html

2.19 Other submissions have suggested that conventional medical scientists and practitioners are inherently biased against CAM. Sir Iain Chalmers, Director of the UK Cochrane Centre, suggests: "Many in the 'orthodox' medical world remain either sceptical about the desirability of this trend [towards increasing use of CAM] or hostile to it. This scepticism seems to result partly from unwillingness within the 'orthodox' mainstream to apply a single evidential standard when assessing the effects of healthcare" (P 223).

2.20 Medical training is now taking full account of many aspects of healthcare, including much of what CAM regards as important, with an increased emphasis on behavioural science, communication skills, counselling, patient-doctor interaction and patient-orientated practice and partnership. And many doctors, despite constraints of time and unremitting pressure, practise holistic medicine. Mr Wainwright Churchill, a traditional acupuncturist and Chinese herbal medicine practitioner from whom we received evidence, pointed out that this pragmatic approach to evaluating CAM satisfies those who see advantages in CAM therapies but believe their theoretical frameworks are invalid (P 256).

2.21 We have been told that even some CAM disciplines with reasonable proof of efficacy are not yet being incorporated into NHS practice. Like Sir Iain Chalmers, mentioned above, other witnesses have suggested there is a non-pragmatic, deep-seated prejudice held by some members of the conventional scientific establishment against the entire CAM field and its philosophy. Other evidence has, however, suggested that such prejudice is diminishing steadily. And it is equally the case that the evident hostility felt towards conventional medicine by some CAM practitioners has had dangerous consequences in delaying unacceptably life-saving conventional treatment. Many such practitioners have in the past shunned the conventional scientific emphasis on rigorous testing and denied the need for research 'because I know it works', or because they believe testing procedures are biased and neglect to measure important aspects of the CAM encounter (see Chapter 7). However, these extreme attitudes do seem to be changing, with better communication between the practitioners of the two fields and moves towards integrated medicine.

2.22 Evidence received during the course of our Inquiry has made it clear that many conventional scientists and doctors believe that the procedures, principles and efficacy of CAM should be scrutinised by the methods of conventional science. Many CAM practitioners resent this attitude, believing it to be indicative of a lack of understanding and sympathy towards CAM within mainstream healthcare. The fact that CAM and conventional medicine approach health from different perspectives, has caused antipathy between the two sides. Conventional medicine accuses CAM practitioners of being "anti-scientific" and illogical and many CAM practitioners accuse conventional medicine of taking an over-simplistic view of illness and of neglecting important areas of a patient's experience. However, in recent years, many practitioners in conventional and complementary medicine have begun to take a more open-minded view. In the conventional medical profession there is increasing support for the view that medical practitioners and other healthcare professionals should begin to work with CAM practitioners. Evidence from the Academy of Medical Royal Colleges confirmed that "pressure is now coming on the medical profession, to look around them and see all other practitioners and make sure it all works well for the patient" (Q 299). Integrated healthcare programmes are thus beginning to develop.

2.23 During our Inquiry we visited the Marylebone Health Centre which is an inner London NHS GP practice where GPs and CAM therapists work together for the benefit of the patient and where, through their collaboration, they have gained increasing respect for each other's approaches (see Appendix 4). We have been made aware of many similar collaborative ventures within the NHS, both in primary and secondary care: this will be discussed in Chapter 9. Agreement is also being reached over approaches to research. The different philosophical approaches may make it hard to design trials with methods that are acceptable to both conventional and CAM practitioners, but as Chapter 7 discusses, novel methods that are acceptable to conventional science and that take into account concerns of both paradigms are being developed. Finally, how important it is to understand and agree on the mechanisms of actions behind a treatment will be considered in Chapter 4.

CHAPTER 3: PATIENT SATISFACTION, THE ROLE OF THE THERAPIST AND
THE PLACEBO RESPONSE

Patient Satisfaction

3.1 Much of our evidence, including that given by the Consumers' Association and the Patients' Association, has suggested that patients' satisfaction with their CAM treatment is high and is likely to account in part for a significant proportion of the high level of CAM use. During the course of our Inquiry the Committee met several patients of CAM practitioners (at the Marylebone Health Centre and at the Southampton Centre for Complementary Health Studies – see Appendices 4 and 5), all of whom expressed high levels of satisfaction with the CAM treatment they had received. We also received many written letters of support for CAM by patients. We did not in fact hear directly from any patients who were unhappy with treatment they had received from a CAM practitioner. The high satisfaction shown by CAM patients suggests that the reasons given (in paras 1.24-1.28) for accessing CAM are largely justified in the event, and the conditions for which they seek help are indeed often relieved, as Zollman and Vickers stated in an article in the *British Medical Journal* last year[16].

3.2 During the our visit to Exeter University (see Appendix 3), Professor Edzard Ernst referred to a project his department had carried out, which compared satisfaction levels with CAM to satisfaction levels with conventional medicine, amongst arthritis sufferers who had experienced both types of treatment[17]. This work suggested that many CAM therapists were more friendly, spent more time with the patient and were more forthcoming with information on the treatment and the disease. Some patients also perceived CAM as giving slightly more efficacious treatments.

3.3 Evidence we heard from the Consumers' Association identified several reasons for high patient satisfaction with CAM. They concluded that patients appreciate CAM's emphasis on a person's overall well-being, and also suggested that the CAM consultation may be more satisfying to patients as it is longer, and CAM practitioners tend to have very good communication skills which put patients at ease. The Consumers' Association had conducted a survey in 1997 which showed that for therapies such as yoga, aromatherapy, massage and reflexology, people experience general life-style benefits just from the experience of taking part in the therapy (Q 829).

3.4 Submissions from the Royal College of Physicians (P 189) and the UK Cochrane Centre (P 223) both suggest that CAM consultations not only take more time, but are more thorough and more detailed than conventional medical consultations, especially in primary care. They also tend to include active listening techniques and demonstrate interest in the whole of the patient's life, not just in their physical health. Such factors may well contribute to higher levels of patient satisfaction with their treatment. Increasing pressures on conventional medical practitioners in an understaffed NHS are felt to be an important contributory factor.

3.5 Zollman and Vickers[18] gave several explanations for the popularity of CAM. It was suggested that the "...specific effects of particular therapies obviously account for a proportion of patient satisfaction, but many patients also value some of the general attributes of complementary medicine." These 'attributes' include those mentioned above but also add: the attention to personality and personal experience, the increased amount of patient involvement and choice, the increased levels of hope often provided by the holistic approach, the more human experience of healthcare (which comes from the increased amount of touch and 'low tech' equipment used in CAM), and the fact that CAM often specialises in dealing with ill-defined symptoms that conventional medicine sometimes is unable, or unwilling, to tackle. Finally they suggest that the holistic approach often provides a means of making sense of illness in a context that is more understandable and personally relevant to the patient.

3.6 HealthWatch (P 123) has suggested that one reason for patient satisfaction is that most CAM practitioners work in private practice and therefore have more time and greater resources with which to help their patients. Several CAM practitioners and HealthWatch (P 123) propose that CAM may function better in the private sector, as the experience of paying for healthcare increases patients' involvement in their own recovery and provides additional motivation. This may lead to greater treatment compliance and a greater degree of satisfaction.

---

[16]   Zollman, C. & Vickers, A. (1999) 'ABC of Complementary Medicine: Complementary Medicine & the Patient'. *British Medical Journal;* 319 (1999) 1486-1489.

[17]   Resch, K., Hill, S. & Ernst, E. (1997) 'Use of Complementary Therapies by Individuals with Arthritis'. *Clinical Rheumatology;* 16:371.5.

[18]   Zollman, C. & Vickers, A. (1999) (*Op.cit.*).

3.7 Looked at altogether this evidence identifies several factors considered by many to contribute to patient satisfaction with CAM. The holistic approach of CAM, the individual emphasis, the greater time spent on patients by practitioners, were all very popular reasons given by witnesses for patient satisfaction. However, Dr George Lewith, head of the Centre for Complementary Health Studies in Southampton told us, during our visit, that no empirical evidence has shown that issues such as time account wholly for patient satisfaction. Therefore, no firm conclusions on the reasons behind patient satisfaction with CAM can be drawn until studies are conducted on this issue. We assume that time is an important factor but it is also likely that quality and not just quantity is important in relation to consultations. Although patient satisfaction may be a component of well-being and a marker of health itself, it is not necessarily a clear reflection of a treatment's clinical efficacy. The placebo effect can have a large role in patient satisfaction as can many of the factors discussed above. The role of patient satisfaction as a component of efficacy will be considered later in this report (see paras 4.24-4.27) as will the role of the placebo effect in CAM and conventional medicine (see paras 3.19 – 3.34).

Patient Dissatisfaction

3.8 Some of the areas identified above as strengths of CAM are fields which conventional medicine, as currently practised, has difficulty in handling. Constraints on time and other pressures on the NHS, and the reliance on drug prescribing in conventional medicine, have eroded the time patients spend with doctors and has tended to lead to a forced discussion of 'the problem' rather than also embracing the context in which the problem needs to be considered. This can lead to the patient feeling that the doctor has not paid him or her much attention or taken time to understand fully what is wrong with them.

3.9 The Consumers' Association suggested that one reason patients turn to CAM is the welcome that they receive from CAM as opposed to conventional medicine. The NHS has long waiting lists for out-patient appointments in secondary care, and there is a common impression among patients, even in primary care (with, on average, seven-minute consultations throughout the NHS) that the doctor's time is precious and must not be wasted. In comparison, CAM therapists are numerous and often easy to access; they are very welcoming to patients, positively encouraging long consultations. The Consumers' Association also suggest that some CAM therapists work in more pleasant environments, and patients appreciate the better, and often more relaxing, quality of their surroundings. The Consumers' Association made the point that people hate to give up hope of getting better when they are ill; therefore if conventional medicine fails to provide a cure, they are likely to look elsewhere in the hope of finding a solution (Q 828).

3.10 Patients are also becoming increasingly aware of, and concerned about, the side-effects of conventional medical treatment, and particularly those of potent drugs. This is a problem the Faculty of Homeopathy, which represents medical practitioners who also practise homeopathy, told us they were very well aware of (P 81). The risk of iatrogenic[19] disease is therefore another reason why patients may try to find alternatives to conventional therapy.

3.11 It can be concluded that there are some factors in conventional medicine that lead patients to turn elsewhere to find the type of treatment to which they aspire. The Consumers' Association evidence points out that it is not invariably a matter of patients turning their back on one mode of treatment and replacing it with another. They suggest that the Government and the NHS are currently emphasising self-treatment of minor ailments, if only because of the inadequate numbers of doctors in all branches of medicine, and patients are increasingly taking on their rights and responsibilities and are choosing treatments that they feel are right for them. Therefore it is likely that the increased use of CAM is a result of patients using a 'pick and mix' combination of treatments rather than a sign of rejection of one school of medicine for another (Q 828). The Astin Survey, discussed above (see para 1.24) would appear to support this conclusion.

3.12 Whether this is true or not it is clear that conventional medicine as presently practised may lack something so that some patients are left feeling that not all their needs have been met. This factor, coupled with developments such as the Internet and the increased emphasis of consumer involvement in all service areas, has led to patients being increasingly aware of their options and responsibilities.

The Role of the Therapist

3.13 Many of our witnesses, both from conventional and from complementary backgrounds, have suggested that the consultation styles of CAM practitioners may play a large role in determining patients' satisfaction with CAM treatment. Many of our witnesses also cited difficulties with the

---

[19] The Oxford English Dictionary defines iatrogenic disease as "Med. (of an illness or symptoms) induced in a patient as a result of a physician's words or action".

relationship between conventional practitioners and their patients, as well as the limited amount of time conventional practitioners have for their patients, as reasons why many patients are turning to CAM. However, little work has been done on this topic.

3.14 During the course of our Inquiry several witnesses drew our attention to *Complementary Medicine: A Research Perspective*[20]. This book includes a chapter on the consultation styles of conventional and complementary practitioners which reviews the few studies that there are in this area.

3.15 The work of one researcher in this area, Taylor, is reviewed in Vincent & Furnham's book. Taylor's work investigates the changing nature of the conventional medical encounter in the United Kingdom. Taylor suggests that in the last thirty years the consumer movement, the increased sense of entitlement and general demands for professional reform and accountability, have put pressure for democratisation and attention to customer service on the medical profession. However Taylor's work suggests the medical profession has resisted change and that there has in fact been a deterioration in the customer service side of the medical encounter. Several reasons are suggested for this:

- The increased threat of malpractice suits has made doctors more cautious and less relaxed with patients.

- There are fewer general practitioners and more specialists so a long-term doctor-patient relationship is less likely.

- Patients find changing doctors and getting second opinions a struggle and so feel they have no 'exit' option within the medical encounter.

- Patients feel doctors insist on clinical autonomy and they perceive a refusal to share information.

- Increased administration within the health service makes patients feel as if more attention is being paid to 'processing' them than appreciating their individual patterns and matching treatment to them.

- Increasing costs and rationing of services has led to feeling that services are being withdrawn.

3.16 These factors are coupled with the fact that, through high-profile medical advances, conventional medicine has acquired great power, prestige and influence, leading to even greater demand for services. This contributes to a vicious circle, whereby patients are demanding more, and feeling as though they are receiving less.

3.17 Vincent & Furnham's book goes on to review the characteristics of the CAM practitioner-patient relationship. They review the work of Kleinman[21] who suggests that although most CAM therapies do not share a common theoretical basis what they do share, which distinguishes them from conventional medicine, is an emphasis on the subjective experience of the patient and a focus on the whole patient, not just the disease. Kleinman suggests that there are several areas where CAM consultation styles may prove more attractive than those of conventional medicine. These are:

- Emphasis on overall experience of illness - CAM therapists often take into account social issues during their assessment of a patient, whereas some conventional medicine increasingly focuses on the individual patient and the specific complaint and bodily organ, or organs, involved. As patients will experience their problem in the context of their family and work etc. and may even see these things as the cause of their problems, they may prefer the CAM approach.

- Simple language - The language of conventional medicine has become increasingly technical and hard for patients to understand. CAM practitioners are more likely to use everyday language.

- Lay explanations - CAM explanations for disease are often easier for a patient to understand than the more technical conventional medical explanations. CAM explanatory models are also more likely to consider factors such as emotional and social factors in disease and so will be concerned with the patient's overall experience. This may lead to circumstances where there is a better fit between patient's view and the views of CAM practitioners.

- Illness without pathology – Patients sometimes feel that something is wrong but are told after a physical examination by a conventional medical practitioner that nothing can be found to support their claims of illness. However, in many cases they continue to feel unwell.

[20] Vincent, C. & Furnham, A. *Complementary Medicine: A Research Perspective* (Chichester; Wiley & Sons; 1997) 119-121.

[21] Kleinman, J. (1980) *as cited in:* Vincent, C. & Furnham, A. (1997) (*Op.cit.*).

Complementary practitioners are often more willing to diagnose and treat such symptoms and to provide an explanation which will be more satisfactory for the patient.

3.18 Another study is discussed in Vincent & Furnham's book, which shows that a doctor's consultative style can have considerable immediate, intermediate and long-term outcomes on patient health. Three communication variables have been found to have importance in the consultation: creating a good interpersonal (trusting, warm, open) relationship; the clear and comprehensible exchange of information; and skill in making treatment-related decisions. The study that identified these variables also identified four major medical outcomes that these variables affect: overall satisfaction; compliance and adherence to a treatment programme; the recall and understanding of exchanged information; final health status; and psychiatric morbidity[22]. This work suggests that the communication styles of CAM therapists, in comparison to conventional therapists, may play a significant role in determining patient satisfaction with CAM. There are two important implications that arise from this. Firstly, CAM research must take into account the potential effects of the patient-practitioner relationship and not side-line it as an incidental factor or a complication in research (see Chapter 7). Secondly, conventional medicine and the NHS may learn from CAM's strengths in this area. It is important to note that many practising medical practitioners possess and are taught exactly those communication skills and appreciation of the emotional and social factors which cause or influence disease, but may be prevented from deploying these skills fully because of pressures and constraints of time. It is widely accepted that some of the most intractable problems which patients present to doctors, often expressed as "illness without pathology" (see above), have a psychological or social basis of which the patient (and sometimes the doctor) may not be fully aware, or which they may be unable to acknowledge.

Placebo Effect

3.19 Psychological factors not only play an important role in giving rise to symptoms but also in determining a patient's response to a treatment. Studies have shown that patient expectations concerning a treatment, patients' experience of the treatment and patients' attitudes towards their healthcare provider can all affect the impact a treatment has. Such factors as these can all be brought together under the term 'the placebo effect'. The placebo effect has been described as the therapeutic impact of 'non-specific' or 'incidental' treatment ingredients, as opposed to the therapeutic impact that can be directly attributed to the specific, characteristic action of the treatment. However, the placebo effect has often in the past had a negative stigma attached to it, and has often been considered either as a nuisance which hampers research, a sign of patient neuroticism, or a sign of clinical quackery.

3.20 The placebo effect is known to permeate all areas of healthcare. Professor Tom Meade of the Royal Society articulated this for us: "...we all recognise the strong placebo effect in, probably, all aspects of medical treatment, whether they are conventional or not" (Q 155). However, it has been suggested by some of our witnesses that the placebo effect may be responsible for much of the apparent benefit of CAM therapies which have no other understandable mechanism of action through which they may affect the body. Before considering this further it is worth considering the complicated history and definition of the placebo effect. Only recently has it begun to be considered in a more positive light.

3.21 The placebo effect is nothing new, nor are attempts to enhance its effect unconventional. In fact the history of conventional medicine has largely been the history of the placebo effect. Vincent & Furnham's book also has a chapter on this subject, written by Phil Richardson who reviews some interesting studies. Most medicines used by doctors up until the 20th Century are now known to be inert, but they were often of exotic origin and thus were often perceived as having magical properties. Even today part of the conventional doctor's armoury may include inert capsules and sugar pills. In fact one study showed that 80 per cent of US hospital clinicians admitted to the occasional use of placebo medicines in routine clinical practice (Gray & Flynn, 1981)[23]. The reasons these doctors gave for this practice were concerned with deflecting the focus of the demanding patient and proving that the symptom thereby reduced was psychogenic and not of organic origin.

3.22 However, some would argue that these reasons demonstrate only a limited knowledge of relevant empirical findings. All treatments, physically active or otherwise, have a psychological impact when administered to a conscious patient. It is possible that this psychological effect should not be considered as a nuisance that hampers research or some kind of fraud, but an essential element of any holistic therapy. It could even be suggested that the placebo effect is a legitimate form of psychotherapy.

---

[22] Ong, de Haes and Lammes, (1995) *as cited in:* Vincent, C. & Furnham, A. (1997) *(Op.cit.)*.

[23] Gray & Flynn (1981) *as cited in:* Vincent, C. & Furnham, A. (1997) *(Op.cit.)*.

3.23 Many studies have been conducted where placebo treatments have been compared to no-treatment controls. Evidence from a wide range of studies indicates that placebo therapies in the context of conventional medicine can provide some relief from a huge range of conditions including allergies, angina, asthma, some forms of cancer, cerebral infarction, depression, diabetes, epilepsy, multiple sclerosis, ulcers and warts. Placebo responses have also been found to vary enormously — from 0 - 100 per cent — even for the same condition[24].

3.24 In the past the placebo effect has often had negative connotations as a worthless by-product of a treatment, notable only in that it complicates research design. As more evidence on this subject becomes available it may be considered that the term placebo effect is unhelpful because it embraces a number of disparate phenomena that are poorly understood. Evidence from placebo studies has provided ammunition to contradict the claim that the placebo effect can be attributed to the patient's wish to please the doctor by reporting symptom relief. Research shows the placebo effect has a measurable effect on objective measures such as blood pressure, post-operative swelling and gastric mobility (Richardson, 1989)[25]. In addition, there is increasing evidence of a neuro-effector mechanism ("mind over matter") which can influence significantly the immune system. In drug action trials there are sometimes even difficulties in differentiating placebos from the active agents that they are being compared with; several studies have shown parallel time-effect curves and dose-response relationships[26].

3.25 Studies in this area clearly show that the psychological impact of any treatment is potentially great. Comparing placebo groups to no-treatment groups does not rule out the possibility that the placebo effect is due to data distortion on the part of therapists, or even the possibility that results are affected by patients with high expectations or a desire to please the doctor. This is because it is very hard to blind patients to the simple fact that they are receiving treatment. However this does not explain changes in objectively measured physiological processes, and thus it seems there is a psychologically-mediated physical effect of most treatments.

3.26 Many studies in this area have looked into whether there are particular patient variables that increase the likelihood that an individual will exhibit the placebo effect. Although such studies have looked into a multitude of factors including sociological factors such as age, gender, ethnicity, educational level and intelligence, and personality factors such as extroversion and suggestibility, they have yielded weak and inconclusive results. It seems that placebo responders cannot be characterised by this type of variable. In fact evidence shows that people who are placebo responders on one occasion may not be on the next: thus it is not an enduring trait. Awareness of the fact that any patient may benefit from the placebo effect might do much to de-stigmatise it as a sign of patient neuroticism.

3.27 There has also been research on which therapies produce the strongest placebo effect. More serious or invasive procedures do seem to have greater placebo properties, with placebo surgery yielding very high positive response rates. Treatments that employ sophisticated technical equipment also enhance the placebo effect. Research on therapist variables has shown that those therapists who exhibit greater interest in their patients, greater confidence in their treatments and higher professional status, whatever their background of training, all appear to promote stronger placebo responses in their patients. This work does not entirely support the view that CAM's effects may be due to the placebo effect. CAM is not generally highly invasive, nor does it tend to involve highly sophisticated technical equipment. However, CAM therapists do seem to exhibit great interest in their patients and confidence in their treatments. It is also possible that the almost "magical" approach of some complicated and unusual therapies may have a similar effect to highly sophisticated technologies in inducing wonder in patients.

3.28 It is important to consider the possible modes of action through which the placebo effect may operate. Professor Patrick Bateson, Vice President of the Royal Society, explained how psychological factors might affect physical health: "...when somebody suffers chronic stress, bereavement or loses a job, under those conditions they are much more prone to disease and more likely to get cancer, and it is now believed that this is because of suppression of the immune system, which is constantly cleaning up bacteria and viruses and also cleaning up cells which are cancerous cells. So if you do the opposite of that and give a patient some reassurance, and if they are given a treatment which they believe in, then this will enhance the immune response - it will remove the stress which is causing the immune response to be suppressed - and so that may be one rather powerful mechanism by which the placebo effect works" (Q 155). However it is widely accepted that the exact mechanisms of action are as yet not well understood. Professor Timothy Shallice of the Academy of Medical Sciences was one of

---

[24] Ross & Olson (1982) *as cited in:* Vincent, C. & Furnham, A. (1997) *(Op.cit.)*.

[25] Richardson (1989) *as cited in:* Vincent, C. & Furnham, A. (1997) *(Op.cit.)*.

[26] Ross & Olson (1982) *as cited in:* Vincent, C. & Furnham, A. (1997) *(Op.cit.)*.

several witnesses who acknowledged this gap in our knowledge: "We would agree that the placebo effect is not fully understood, but this is because essentially the higher cognitive functions in general are not very well understood and the placebo effect operates through belief and a whole series of mechanisms on the body in general through the central nervous system" (P 1403).

3.29 Despite a lack of understanding of the exact mechanisms through which the placebo effect may operate, research clearly shows that the effect exists and can have a significant impact on health. This work has important implications for anyone who has identified a therapy which appears to be efficacious but which does not have a clearly identified mode of action and it is important that all research on such therapies takes account of the placebo effect.

3.30 Research in this area, and evidence we have heard, suggests that it may be over-simplistic, when evaluating physical treatment methods, to ask whether the treatment is a placebo or not. The more pertinent question will often be: "In what proportion may the effects of this treatment be accounted for by psychologically-mediated, as opposed to direct physically-mediated, changes?"[27] In the absence of direct evidence from placebo-controlled double-blind trials[28] it is proper to regard any new or unusual form of treatment as potentially a form of psychotherapy. This is the reason why the debate over the need for randomised controlled trials has become a central debate in the CAM world

3.31 We have also considered the implications of finding that any particular CAM therapy relies largely on the placebo effect and has little or no treatment-specific effect. Several of our witnesses have suggested this is a very important question. Professor Tom Meade of the Royal Society summed up this sentiment: "I think the important question is that if a CAM is claiming that it has a specific value for a particular condition, then it does have to be able to show that there is a treatment-specific effect over and above the placebo effect. I think that is important because, first of all, a lot of CAM is practised in private practice at the moment, and people...are entitled to know how they are spending their money. I think it is also important from the health service's point of view, as various trusts and general practitioners take CAMs up in increasing numbers (Q 155).

3.32 If a treatment makes people feel better, whether that be through treatment specific effects or the placebo effect, then it could be considered as being worthwhile. In fact, as the placebo effect is not just an imagined experience but can positively improve objective biological measures of health, then a treatment which enhanced such an effect could even be considered worth attaining in its own right. As well as stressing the need to prove treatment-specific effects Professor Patrick Bateson, giving evidence with Professor Tom Meade for the Royal Society, acknowledged that sometimes the placebo effect may be worth attaining in its own right.

3.33 However, the idea that the placebo effect might be something worth using as a treatment was not a majority opinion, and Professor Timothy Shallice of the Academy of Medical Sciences suggested that there is probably little justification for supporting the wider advocacy of any technique that relies on the placebo effect within the NHS "...since it depends so critically on the particular beliefs of that particular person at that particular time" (P 1403).

3.34 Professor Peter Lachmann of the Academy of Medical Sciences elaborated on why treatments which work through the placebo effect are not worth using as a treatment: "...it is not surprising that therapies which have no pharmacological basis but which affect mental state can stimulate the secretion of endogenous opioids and other mediators that affect lymphocytes because they also carry the relevant receptors. The fact remains that methods of doing just this (for example jogging) are not used for treating visceral diseases, nor are similar claims made for them. That immune cells can be affected by neurological mechanisms is neither unconventional nor terribly surprising" (Q 1413).

---

[27] Richardson, P. (1997) *as cited in* Vincent, C. & Furnham, A. (*Op. cit.*).

[28] Trials in which neither the practitioner nor the patient are aware of which treatment is being administered. In single-blind trials only the patient is unaware of which treatment is being administered.

CHAPTER 4: EVIDENCE

4.1 There are several types of evidence that it is desirable to obtain before a therapy is advocated:

- Evidence that the therapy is efficacious above and beyond the placebo effect (see paras 3.19 – 3.34);

- Evidence that the therapy is safe;

- Evidence that the therapy is cost-effective;

- Evidence concerning the mechanism of action of the therapy.

Methods available for obtaining such evidence will be discussed in Chapter 7 : Research.

Evidence for Efficacy?

4.2 The conclusions from research into the efficacy of the various CAMs are outside the remit of this report. However, it is necessary to understand the general state of the CAM evidence base, in order to consider what type of evidence needs to be collected and to understand why CAM's claims often cause controversy.

4.3 CAM has been criticised by some witnesses for not having scientific evidence to back its claims. The Academy of Medical Sciences (P 1) told us that they are concerned that many CAM practitioners do not take a 'scientific' approach to treatment. They suggest that whereas conventional medicine makes efforts to conduct rigorous research, and changes its clinical practice when new information is discovered, CAM practitioners are more likely to stick to their belief systems despite any negative evidence that may emerge. This is one reason the Academy of Medical Sciences uses to explain why CAM lacks an adequate evidence base to convince them, as conventional scientists, of its claims. This is a controversial statement, and as discussed in para 2.19, Sir Iain Chalmers, Director of the UK Cochrane Centre, suggested that conventional medicine is biased against CAM and conventional medical practitioners and scientists are likely to require lower standards of proof for conventional medical treatments then they do for CAM (P 225). Nevertheless, as we concluded in para 2.7, we are satisfied that there is at present no credible evidence base to support the value of any of the therapies that we list in our Group 3.

4.4 The Department of Health summed up their opinion of the evidence base for CAM by saying that "Evidence for CAM in the form of research has been criticised as being inadequate, and there is some justification in this claim" (P 101). This is a controversial area, as the definition of an adequate evidence base varied across our witnesses. Some CAM practitioners have claimed that a history of safe and apparently successful traditional use is enough evidence to justify advocating the use of their particular therapy. However, most of our witnesses with a conventional medical or scientific background have asserted that, in order for CAM therapies to be more widely accepted, it is important that they have a critical mass of scientifically-controlled evidence to support their claims; and that at the moment most of CAM lacks such evidence. Many of our conventional medical witnesses have suggested that, since much of conventional medicine is required to undergo rigorous trials to justify its use, no less should be expected of CAM. But even this view is controversial as some of the CAM advocates we have heard from have suggested that much of conventional medicine lacks a rigorously tested evidence base, and that to require one of CAM is to operate a double standard. In fact, the Department of Health followed their statement that there was some justification behind the claim that the CAM evidence base was inadequate, by acknowledging that the same could be said for some conventional medicine. It is our view that most modern conventional therapies are backed by scientific evidence. It is in the case of some of the older and traditional treatments surviving from the past (such as cold 'cures' and 'tonics') where evidence is, like the evidence for much of CAM, lacking.

4.5 There are two notable weaknesses of the evidence base for CAM that at present exists. One is that in most of these areas little research is being done, and the second is that the few studies which have been completed are given disproportionate weight. It is worth considering this second feature in some detail. Some CAMs have embarked upon research in order to build up an evidence base. All the therapies that we have included in Group 1 either have done, or are working on, rigorous trials to test their claims. However, one or two studies with positive results in support of their claims for efficacy are not enough. It must be remembered that with a statistical significance of $p<.05$[29] (the commonly accepted level of significance), one in twenty studies of any procedure will show a possible significant effect; hence a few positive results with small effects are not yet enough to prove a therapy's efficacy, nor to justify its wider provision.

---

[29]   A significance level of $p<.05$ means that there is a probability of less than 5% that the results a trial has produced could occur by chance.

4.6 Another problem with the way existing studies are used is that many old studies are recycled again and again through reviews and meta-analyses[30]. There are some doubts about the usefulness and validity of the results of meta-analysis. Professor Peter Lachmann, on behalf of the Academy of Medical Sciences, told us: "Meta-analysis is a highly contentious but very important issue and is subject to all sorts of problems, of which comparable design, selective publication of positive against negative results and various other problems are well-known. Not all meta-analyses should be afforded the same weight" (Q 1411). This problem highlights the need for more original work, involving well-designed clinical trials, to be done on CAM disciplines.

4.7 The importance of evidence of efficacy is less clear than the importance of evidence of safety. Many witnesses have suggested that if a person feels that a therapy is helpful to them and can be shown not to be harming them, then it is not necessary for there to be statistically valid research supporting its claims. But the question then arises as to whether such a treatment should be made available at public expense. The role of patient satisfaction in evaluating therapies will be considered in paragraphs 4.24 – 4.27.

4.8 One argument that has been repeated to us is that the existence of evidence which supports a therapy's claims is of secondary importance, provided that patients are aware of whether there is any evidence or not. Consumer bodies such as Patient Concern (P 166) believe that treating a patient with a therapy that lacks evidence of efficacy is not wrong if the patient is happy with the treatment, as long as he or she knows that there is no definitive proof of efficacy and has not been led to believe that the treatment will definitely work. They call for strong measures to be taken against practitioners who mislead patients with false claims of evidence of efficacy.

4.9 Another issue to consider in this area is how much evidence there is to support the claims of other healthcare interventions so as to consider the position of CAM in context. The Medicines Control Agency require evidence of efficacy (and of quality and safety) before licensing any new pharmaceutical product. However, the British Dental Association (P 35) gave evidence suggesting that much of clinical dental practice has a weak evidence base. We have also heard evidence concerning several commonly used conventional medical treatments that have a long history of use but little research evidence to support such use. Examples include the use of electro-convulsive therapy for the treatment of depression and cervical and uterine curettage for treating dysfunctional uterine bleeding.

4.10 However, the Institute of Biology (P 125), suggest that if health practitioners are to be held liable for their services to their patients then the medicines they prescribe must be proven to be efficacious.

4.11 There are complications in this area beyond simply evaluating the importance of evidence of efficacy. Many submissions from CAM representatives, as well as the submission from the NHS Confederation (P 144), claim that, for some forms of CAM in some situations, there is already evidence of efficacy. Therefore they suggest that the lack of mainstream acceptance and the slow NHS uptake must be due to other factors. The NHS Confederation claims CAM has suffered from 'unscientific prejudice' from the scientific orthodoxy; however most conventional medicine submissions deny this, and reiterate the argument that a few positive studies should not be given too much weight and do not constitute a critical mass of evidence (para 4.5). In particular, positive trials of homeopathic treatment in allergic disorders have not yet convinced many conventional practitioners. Specifically, trials at the Glasgow Homeopathic Hospital, demonstrating benefit in the treatment of asthma and allergic rhinitis with homeopathic remedies, are thought by some independent observers to need larger and longer trials for confirmation of the perceived effects.

4.12 Beyond these general points the diversity of CAM therapies is such that our comments must be related to the three groups of disciplines that we have listed in Box 1.

4.13 Of the therapies in Group 1 we were made aware of good evidence of the efficacy of osteopathy and chiropractic[31]. Indeed, they appear to be somewhat more effective than the manipulative techniques employed by conventional physiotherapists. There is also scientific evidence of the efficacy of acupuncture, notably for pain relief and the treatment of nausea[32]. The evidence for the efficacy of herbal medicine is mixed. Many herbs have established activities while others do not;

---

[30] Meta-analysis is the combination of data from several studies to produce a single estimate. From the statistical point of view, meta-analysis is a straightforward application of multi-factorial methods. If there are several studies of the same thing with each giving an estimate of an effect, the meta-analysis provides a common estimate representative of all the work.

[31] See: Vincent, C. & Furnham, A. (1997) (*Op.cit.*), 'The quality of medical information and the evaluation of acupuncture, osteopathy and chiropractic'.

[32] British Medical Association. *The evidence base of acupuncture* in: *Acupuncture: efficacy, safety practice*. Harwood Academic Publishers, London (2000); pp 7 – 37.

among those which are active many are claimed to have numerous other actions for which evidence is lacking. Many powerful drugs used in conventional medicine are of herbal origin, such as morphine derived from the poppy, or digoxin from the foxglove. Problems sometimes arise when mixtures of herbs are used. Even when these are of proven efficacy it may be difficult to identify the active ingredient or ingredients and some preparations may be difficult to standardise and control. In the case of homeopathy, although it is covered by a separate Act of Parliament, we were not able to find any totally convincing evidence of its efficacy. Nevertheless, we accept that there is anecdotal evidence of benefit from homeopathic remedies in animals, where presumably a placebo effect is less significant. Much more research is needed.

4.14 Of the therapies in Group 2 there are many claims of efficacy, usually for a limited range of ailments. We have not examined each in detail. We see many of these complementary therapies as inducing relaxation and a sense of well-being so as presumably to stimulate the immune response, as in the placebo effect. Many are greatly appreciated for the comfort they provide to terminally ill patients.

4.15 We find no convincing evidence of efficacy for any of the remedies in Groups 3a or 3b, but we did not carry out a detailed examination.

4.16 Evidence for the efficacy of the treatment itself is not the only important factor. The Royal Society of Edinburgh (P 212) makes the point that evidence of the validity of diagnostic procedures is as important as evidence supporting efficacy of a treatment. **Diagnostic procedures must be reliable and reproducible and more attention must be paid to whether CAM diagnostic procedures as well as CAM therapies, have been scientifically validated. We agree that this is an issue that should always be kept in mind when doing research in this area.**

4.17 More research is needed on the efficacy of most CAMs. In the case of therapies which possess research evidence, but whose practitioners believe that conventional scientific views are standing in the way of their acceptance, it would be constructive if a body such as the National Institute for Clinical Excellence (NICE) could evaluate such evidence as exists. (NICE did point out that topics they enquire into are determined by the Department of Health and are selected against a framework of the State's priorities for the NHS (Q 1839). However, they did acknowledge that, in their view, such subjects may be suitable for appraisals). It would also help if such bodies made sure that on their evaluation committees were doctors and scientists who were aware of CAM's intricacies, philosophy and research (see Chapter 7).

4.18 **In our opinion any discipline whose practitioners make specific claims for being able to treat specific conditions should have evidence of being able to do this above and beyond the placebo effect. This is especially true for therapies which aim to be available on the NHS and aim to operate as an alternative to conventional medicine, specifically therapies in Group 1. The therapies in our Groups 3a and 3b also aim to operate as an alternative to conventional medicine, and have sparse, or non-existent, evidence bases. Those therapies in our Group 2 which aim to operate as an adjunct to conventional medicine and mainly make claims in the area of relaxation and stress management are in lesser need of proof of treatment-specific effects but should control their claims according to the evidence available to them.**

Evidence for Safety

4.19 Evidence that a therapy has few, if any, significant adverse effects and will not cause avoidable harm must be considered important in all medicine, including CAM. However, there are two potential complications which confound this seemingly simple statement:

- What level of safety should be demanded?

- What type of evidence of safety is acceptable?

4.20 In determining what level of safety should be sought, the risk/benefit ratio of the therapy in question must be considered. If the potential benefits of a therapy are likely to be very significant, or even life-saving, then the level of risk a patient may be willing to take with the therapy is likely to be higher than the level of risk they are willing to accept for the benefit of temporary symptom relief or the cure of a minor complaint. Another consideration is whether the risks a therapy may possess are inherent or can be minimised through proper regulation of its practitioners. For example we received some evidence about the risks of acupuncture causing pneumothorax due to a needle being inserted into the pleural cavity; however if practitioners are properly trained and well-regulated this risk is minimised. In determining what evidence of safety is acceptable it is important to consider what weight should be given to a history of safe traditional use. Within CAM such evidence is common and is often given reasonable weight by CAM advocates and to a certain extent by policy-makers. For example there are exemptions from licensing in the Medicines Acts for natural remedies of traditional use, and a third category of medicines, which will include traditional-use herbal medicines, is being examined by the European Union (see Chapter 5).

4.21 There is no doubt that many CAM therapies are very safe, as compared to many new powerful conventional remedies. This is often used as an argument for approving the increasing use of CAM, but it must be remembered that the use of a "safe" CAM remedy to treat a serious or potentially lethal disease, so that the use of conventional preparations with proven efficacy is denied, is of course a real danger.

4.22 Several submissions we received suggest that minimum standards of safety need to be defined and widely disseminated in order to protect the public. The British Holistic Medical Association have suggested that such work should be carried out by NICE and the Commission for Health Improvement (CHI) who should then issue national guidelines.

4.23 The evidence that we received from almost all the different therapies indicated that at the point of diagnosis, if the practitioners thought that their treatment would not work, they would refer their patients to a conventional medical practitioner. We were encouraged by this sentiment, even though it was not universal.

Patient Satisfaction As Evidence For Efficacy

4.24 We have heard many conflicting opinions on the idea that high levels of patient satisfaction could be used as evidence for a therapy's efficacy. It has been argued by some that such satisfaction is very important. The International Federation of Reflexologists (P 129) suggest that evaluation of patient satisfaction is particularly important in CAM because much of CAM emphasises patients' participation in the therapy and evaluation of its effects. Many other witnesses have asserted that although patient satisfaction has its place it is not sufficient to justify accepting that a therapy works so that objective rather than subjective evidence is needed. The Academy of Medical Sciences explained why this may be: "It needs to be emphasised that patient satisfaction is not in itself a sufficient estimate of clinical benefit. While it is very important that patients be satisfied with the efforts made on their behalf, it is at least equally important that they should obtain objective benefit. The two do not always go together. For example, patients with peripheral vascular disease, if they go to a practitioner who allows them to continue smoking will show a high patient satisfaction although their outcome will be poor. In contrast, if they are made to stop smoking they are likely to be dissatisfied but their outcome will be much better" (p 286).

4.25 NICE, who have been charged with the responsibility of evaluating the evidence for different NHS treatments over the coming years, also express concern about the validity of anecdotal evidence such as patient satisfaction. Professor Sir Michael Rawlins, Chairman of NICE, told us: "Anecdote, by and large, is not a very reliable method for determining efficacy and 2000 years of medicine demonstrate the fragility of anecdote as a basis for practising medicine" (Q 1833).

4.26 One point that most of our witnesses have agreed upon is that patient experience is important enough to warrant patients being involved in the appraisal of therapies. NICE have made moves towards incorporating patients' views into their appraisals. Mr Andrew Dillon, Chief Executive of NICE, told us: "In the process we have established we invited nationally-based patient advocate groups to make submissions into our individual appraisals. So we have a written statement of their assessment of, as far as they understand it, the patient's perspective of the disease, and if it is an intervention which is currently in use in the NHS, their understanding of the patient's experience of using that intervention in the management of their illness. We also invite patient advocates to join the appraisal committee meetings themselves" (Q 1843).

4.27 In conclusion, patient satisfaction has its place as part of the evidence base for CAM but its position is complicated, as Sir Michael Rawlins, explained: "The difficulty, of course, is that very often the anecdotal evidence relates to conditions where there is fluctuation in the clinical course and people who start an intervention at a time when there is a natural resolution of the disease, very understandably, are likely to attribute cause and effect when it may not be. But, on the other hand, there are some anecdotes that are quite clearly important." Therefore, ideally studies should include patient satisfaction as one of a number of measures in evaluating a treatment, but it alone cannot be taken as a proof or otherwise of a treatment's efficacy or as evidence to justify provision.

Evidence About Mechanisms of Action

4.28 The position of therapies without a scientifically plausible mechanism of action (e.g. healing and homeopathy) needs to be considered. If there is no scientifically plausible mechanism through which a treatment may work in the human body, can the use of such a therapy be justified? Should such therapies be considered a product of the placebo effect enhanced by "tender loving care" or should consideration be given to the possibility that they may have explanations not yet understood by modern science? (The role of the placebo effect is discussed in paras 3.19-3.34.)

4.29 Many of our witnesses have argued that if there is evidence for efficacy then it is not necessary to understand exactly how the effect is achieved, and we agree. This is, indeed, the position with several conventional therapies. Professor Sir Michael Rawlins explained that in NICE's search for clinical excellence, it is evidence of efficacy and not the mechanism of action that is prioritised: "I do not mind and I do not think the Institute minds whether it understands how a treatment works or not. I do not understand how many treatments do work, and this is after 35 years as a pharmacologist, but what we do like is good evidence that they do whatever they claim to do" (Q 1833).

4.30 However, despite these arguments, the opposite view is that if a therapy has no plausible mechanism of action then spending research money on it and providing patients with access to it is likely to be a waste of resources. It is worth considering this argument in more detail, by asking two distinct questions:

- Should mechanisms of action be plausible before research into the efficacy of a therapy is funded?

- Should mechanisms of action be understood before access to a therapy is provided?

4.31 It is of course true that many treatments have been used for a long time without understanding their mechanisms of action and only now are possible explanations for how they work coming to light. Professor Lesley Rees, a Trustee of FIM, used acupuncture as a case in point. Acupuncture is traditionally said to work through affecting energy meridians that according to Traditional Chinese medicine circulate around each person. This explanation is not congruent with current scientific thought and if an understanding of mechanisms of action were considered of paramount importance doctors should have shunned acupuncture years ago. Now, however, other possible mechanisms, which are more amenable to modern scientific thought (e.g. concerning the effect on the central nervous system and the stimulation of endorphin receptors), are being discovered and evidence for acupuncture's efficacy is growing. As Professor Lesley Rees summed up: "…acupuncture has been used for thousands of years, yet there was no real information about how it might work and I think it would be fair to say that it would have been terrible if the benefits of acupuncture had not been appreciated and used over all the years because we did not have any real understanding of perhaps some of the mechanisms about how they work" (Q 77).

4.32 In terms of research Professor Tom Meade from the Royal Society told us that "…the distinction between the effect and the explanation for the effect is central, and you do not need to believe in the explanation in order to believe in the effect" (Q 181). Therefore, "…it would be perfectly possible for a funding body to allow a bit of research to go forward even though the theoretical backdrop is totally irrelevant to whether the treatment works or not. I think probably what we will see now, increasingly, is applications for funds which simply say 'There is good reason to think there is an effect here and we want to study that. We are going to use these methods which are well attested.' And if everyone agrees that then, if this works out, it will reduce the ambiguity of the effectiveness of this particular treatment" (Q 181).

4.33 A reason for funding efficacy studies of therapies without a plausible mechanism of action is that research into that area can help elucidate routes through which mechanisms of action might work. Professor Meade explained: "…I think it is possible, in some circumstances, that the result of the trial – in other words that something is effective – will actually then give clues as to studying the mechanisms. Equally, if it is not effective then it is beginning to exclude possible explanations as well" (Q 181).

4.34 However, there is an alternative view, articulated by Professor Lewis Wolpert, a fellow of the Academy of Medical Sciences, that: "It is not just efficacy that you should be thinking about. Medicine aims to base itself upon science. Let me tell you what I mean. If you have therapy which you can in no plausible way relate to the behaviour of cells…I personally could not support research in that field" (Q 1404). Based on the limited amount of research funding available in the medical sciences, he suggests that research into therapies such as homeopathy should not be funded: "A liquid which contains no active molecule, which no chemist could plausibly give an account of, is not an area where I would want to invest money. I am sorry: one cannot give up all of chemistry just because one believes homeopathy works" (Q 1404 and 1406). Professor Patrick Bateson, giving evidence on behalf of the Royal Society, summed up this argument by saying the role of mechanisms of action comes into importance because "… the critical thing here is going to be whether there is enough evidence to justify us spending more time and trouble testing the efficacy and safety of treatment" (Q 175).

4.35 The mechanism through which homeopathy may work on the body is a specific case in point, about which we have heard much. Samuel Hahnemann at the turn of the 19th century put forward the "law of similars", claiming that any disease can be treated successfully with minute amounts of a drug which in larger doses gives rise to the same symptoms. Therefore, homeopathy is based on the idea of treating 'like with like' by administering hugely diluted versions of basically dangerous substances, such that a dose given to a patient may not contain even a single molecule of the active principle. Many conventional doctors and scientists cannot accept that infinitesimal dilutions can have any effect on the body.

4.36 The arguments about homeopathy illustrate the weight given to understanding mechanisms of action. The Department of Health explained their position on homeopathy which clearly shows they prioritise safety before anything else and give less weight to issues of scientific plausibility: "In relation to homeopathic medicines, we very much agree that there is uncertainty, or limited evidence, about the specific mechanism whereby homeopathy works. The starting point is that homeopathic medicines as such are very much at the safe end of the spectrum; they are very dilute. Often these substances do not have a clearly measurable effect on the body, which is why the simplified homeopathic registration scheme introduced in 1994 concentrates specifically on safety and quality and not efficacy. We have taken a fairly pragmatic approach: if homeopathy does not harm then it is less important to have an in-depth understanding of its mechanism for effectiveness" (Q 34).

4.37 In terms of research funding for therapies without a scientifically plausible mechanism of action, it seems that opinion within the world of conventional medicine is very divided. However, **we recommend that if a therapy whose mechanism of action is unclear does gain sufficient evidence to support its efficacy, then the NHS and the medical profession should ensure that the public have access to it and its potential benefits.**

4.38 The question of NHS provision for therapies such as homeopathy was answered by the Department of Health by prioritising safety together with consumer choice. On the other hand, as evidence from the Academy of Medical Sciences suggests, the only reason for using therapies such as homeopathy is as a vehicle for the placebo effect to work safely (see paras 3.19 – 3.34). Professor Peter Lachmann told us: "Other effects of homeopathy apropos the placebo effect have already been mentioned and I personally am entirely happy with the idea that homeopathy is a good way of administering a placebo because it is free from harm. I am well aware of the fact that in conventional medicine placebo effects are sometimes produced by the administration of drugs. That is less harmless because all drugs have some side-effects. If drugs are given not for a good purpose but just given to make the patients feel that something is being done for them, then I would entirely agree that a homeopathic preparation, which would produce the same placebo effect without possible harmful side-effects, is to be preferred" (Q 1410).

4.39 The intricate arguments concerning the use of the placebo effect as a therapy were discussed in chapter 3; this does not contradict the argument that safety is a priority, and as long as a therapy is safe, use of any benefits it may bring to patients is justifiable without necessarily understanding its mechanisms. In an era when the Government are hoping that NHS treatments will live up to a standard of evidence set by NICE, we welcome the fact that, as the quotation from Professor Sir Michael Rawlins shows, NICE are willing to accept that a therapy can be efficacious and worth considering even when its mechanisms of action are unclear (see para 4.29).

4.40 It is our opinion that as long as the treatments are known to carry no, or few, adverse effects, it would be against the principle of clinical freedom[33] to prevent patients from having access to therapies which fulfil these criteria and have never been restricted. This is especially the case if the patients believe that such therapies help them and the only argument against them is that an adequate evidence base, derived from controlled trials, does not exist. It is also our opinion that mechanisms of action are of secondary importance to efficacy, a view shared by NICE (Q 1833). We also believe that the principle of clinical freedom should allow therapy with any credible evidence of efficacy the opportunity of validation by further research and the possibility of NHS provision. Any medicine with credible, accepted evidence for efficacy should be available, whatever the controversy over its underlying mechanisms.

---

[33] By "the principle of clinical freedom" we mean the ability of a medical practitioner to exercise freedom of choice in preventing, diagnosing and treating disease within the limits of his or her clinical competence, having regard solely to the welfare and well-being of the individual, and casting all other considerations aside.

CHAPTER 5: REGULATION

5.1 The principal purpose of regulation of any healthcare profession is to protect the public from unqualified or inadequately trained practitioners. The effective regulation of a therapy thus allows the public to understand where to look in order to get safe treatment from well-trained practitioners in an environment where their rights are protected. It also underpins the healthcare professions' confidence in a therapy's practitioners and is therefore fundamental in the development of all healthcare professions. In 1999 the Department of Health commissioned Mr Simon Mills and Ms Sarah Budd at the University of Exeter to produce an information pack on the regulatory prospects for complementary and alternative medicine[34]. This pack states that the purpose of regulation in healthcare is: "To establish a nationwide, professionally determined and independent standard of training, conduct and competence for each profession for the protection of the public and the guidance of employers. To underpin the personal accountability of practitioners for maintaining safe and effective practice and to include effective measures to deal with individuals whose continuing practice presents an unacceptable risk to the public or otherwise renders them unfit to be a registered member of the profession"[35].

5.2 All our witnesses saw that some form of regulation was important; there was widespread consensus that regulation, handled appropriately, had many benefits for the public and the professions. FIM has been heavily involved in promoting better regulation within the various CAM therapies. They explained that: "...in any healthcare profession's therapy group, the quality of care, treatment and patient safety must have the highest priority. In order to achieve this, systems of regulation need to be established and maintained" (P 88). FIM's position is that effective regulation of CAM therapies is central to development in many areas of CAM. Mr Michael Fox, Chief Executive of FIM, told us that "...we do believe at the Foundation that this issue of regulation and working with the complementary professions is fundamental and if that was established properly a lot of things would flow from it" (Q 103).

5.3 In their Regulatory Information Pack (see para 5.1), Budd and Mills also discuss the collateral benefits of regulation. They explain that regulation not only protects the public, but that it results in "...improved professional status and respect; promotion of unity, order, consistency and accountability; greater ability to negotiate with the Government and the NHS; secure therapy-wide benefits such as indemnity insurance; and high common standards for entry and continuing practice"[36].

5.4 The Government view regulation as important. In the Government paper: *The New NHS Modern and Dependable,* it is stated that: "The Government will continue to look to individual health professionals to be responsible for the quality of their own clinical practice. Professional self-regulation must remain an essential element in the delivery of quality patient services"[37]. In May 1998, the then Secretary of State for Health, Frank Dobson, addressed a conference at FIM at which he stated that the Government expected CAM professions "to attain the same standards of professional self-regulation expected of other healthcare professions" (P 105). The Department of Health's evidence also explained their aims for regulation within healthcare: "In matters of regulation, it is the Government's intention to maintain freedom of choice whilst ensuring that appropriate safeguards are in place" (P 101).

5.5 There are two distinct types of regulation, statutory and voluntary. The difference between these two types of regulation will be discussed later in this chapter. However, the type of regulation is probably of less importance than whether the regulation (irrespective of its type) is delivered effectively by a single regulatory body. Professor Edzard Ernst at the Department for Complementary Health Studies, University of Exeter, told us: "The nature of regulation (e.g. statutory regulation or self regulation) seems of secondary importance. What matters is that regulation achieves its primary aim, which is to protect the public. As long as this can be demonstrated, any form of regulation would seem welcome" (P 230).

Current Regulatory Status of CAM Professions

5.6 Mr Michael Fox, Chief Executive of FIM, described the current situation of CAM regulation as variable. He explained that there is "a wide continuum of development" (Q 102). This ranges from

---

[34] Budd, S. & Mills, S. *Regulatory Prospects for Complementary and Alternative Medicine: Information Pack.* University of Exeter (2000), on behalf of the Department of Health.

[35] Budd, S. & Mills, S. (2000) *(Op.cit.).*

[36] Budd, S. & Mills, S. (2000) *(Op.cit.).*

[37] *The New NHS Modern and Dependable*, Department of Health, HSC 1998/228: LAC (98) 32, 8 December 1998.

therapies that are regulated by statute and those that have single voluntary regulatory bodies which operate in a professional manner, to therapies with a multitude of bodies claiming to represent the therapy, none of which has all the features required of an effective regulatory body (see Boxes 4 and 5).

5.7 The primary aim of the University of Exeter survey of the professions of CAM, conducted by Mills and Budd for the Department of Health (see para 1.16), was to establish the current status of United Kingdom professional associations in the field of CAM. The second edition of this study was published earlier this year and so provides an up-to-date overview of this area. Box 2 takes the results of this survey to provide a picture of the current situation regarding the professionalisation of the principal CAM voluntary regulatory bodies in the United Kingdom. Most of the therapies which we have listed in our Groups 3a and 3b (Box 1, Chapter 2), are not included in Box 2 as their size and current state of professional organisation would not, in our view, justify their inclusion or further detailed consideration, since all of them lack a credible evidence base.

Box 2

Status of Some CAM Voluntary Professional Bodies* in the United Kingdom.

Acupuncture — There are five associations representing non-statutory registered health professionals who practise acupuncture. By far the largest of these is the British Acupuncture Council which represents around 2020 acupuncture practitioners and is a result of a unification of five professional groups. The British Acupuncture Council are seen by Mills and Budd as having led the way in establishing verifiable standards of education for their profession. They are associated with the British Acupuncture Accreditation Board which, under an independent chairman, works with the relevant training courses to set out and audit standards of education and training. The British Acupuncture Council have a professional Chief Executive, a core curriculum and a revised code of ethics and practice. They have set up an acupuncture resource centre to encourage undergraduate and post-graduate research. Less is said by Mills and Budd about the other four professional associations in the acupuncture field, two of which failed to give information on how many practitioners they represent.

Alexander Technique — Because Alexander Technique professionals consider themselves not as healthcare professionals treating patients but as teachers teaching students, comparisons with other groups are difficult. Three organisations were identified which represent Alexander Technique Teachers; the largest of these is the Society of Teachers of the Alexander Technique which represents about ninety percent of therapists identified. They are the core group in wider discussions to create a new general council of teachers of the Alexander Technique. Most inter-group differences in this area are historical; however, one group, the Interactive Teaching Methods Association, was set up in 1993 with the view that any single body "should reflect the diversity" in the various training schools: therefore they aspire to be different.

Anthroposophical medicine — There are five bodies that represent Anthroposophical Medicine in the United Kingdom and each represents a different category of statutory practitioner so one is a medical association, one a nursing association, one an art therapists association and another a movement therapists association, while the last represents an approach that is limited to massage. This structure has inhibited moves towards the formation of a common body. Mills and Budd suggest it may be helpful for patients if there were an overarching standards group for all the associations involved.

Aromatherapy — There are twelve organisations representing aromatherapists who practise in the United Kingdom. Eleven of these are members of an umbrella association, the Aromatherapy Organisations Council which provides common codes of ethics and disciplinary procedures and represents the profession in legislative discussions. The one body that does not come within the Aromatherapy Organisations Council's remit is the Institute of Aromatic Medicine which is also the only body to try to use essential oils internally. The Aromatherapy Organisations Council is seen as an early precedent for trying to unite professional groups but there are signs of moves within some of the bodies they represent to establish their own working groups.

Cranio-sacral therapy — There has been an increase in the prominence of these therapy groups, in the wake perhaps of the registration of osteopaths. There are currently three organisations representing people practising these therapies, but recently there have been moves to integrate the cranio-sacral disciplines through the Forum of Cranial and Cranio-Sacral Practitioners.

Healing — There are twelve organisations representing healers practising in the United Kingdom. Five of these are represented by an umbrella body, the Confederation of Healing Organisations. Within this organisation is the British Alliance of Healing Associations which represents twenty-six additional county and church groups. Mills and Budd state that the Confederation has been an effective platform for a great variety of healing organisations and hope that a similar consensus will prevail over the coming years. One of the large professional bodies in this area has suggested that, considering the diversity of standards accepted by the various healing organisations, a two-tier registration with a statutory "professional register" and a voluntary "register" supported by different educational requirements would be appropriate.

Herbal medicine — Mills and Budd found that with the renewed popularity of herbal medicine in recent times there are a number of professional groups, some linked with other cultures or to particular approaches to diagnosis. Many are constituent organisations of the new umbrella body, the European Herbal Practitioners Association. The European Herbal Practitioners Association has declared that it is actively seeking statutory registration for its members and has been in discussions with the Department of Health already.

* *The University of Exeter survey included as "professional bodies" those respondent CAM organisations with professional codes and appropriate corporate status and services to their members and the public. (See also Box 7 for the definition of a profession).*

Box 2 continued

Homeopathy — Mills and Budd point out that homeopathy is practised by two separate groups; medical homeopaths are medically qualified practitioners regulated by the GMC, non-medical homeopaths are professionals who use homeopathy only. Four main bodies representing the non-medical homeopaths were identified. The largest of these is the Society of Homoeopaths. They have formally consulted their membership and committed themselves to pursuing a single register of homeopaths. They have begun to work with the second largest body, the UK Homeopathic Medical Association, and have agreed on National Occupational Standards and created a Joint Meeting of Organisations Representing Professional Homeopaths. Although this is evidence of improved co-ordination among professional homeopaths, there has so far been little communication between these groups and the bodies representing medical homeopaths.

Hypnotherapy — Professional organisation of hypnotherapists is complicated, partly because there is an overlap with the organisations representing psychotherapists who do not consider themselves complementary or alternative and so were not included in Mills and Budd's survey. They identified seventeen bodies representing hypnotherapists; five of these are members of the relatively new umbrella body, the UK Confederation of Hypnotherapy Organisations. Mills and Budd suggest hypnotherapy is an area where consensus has been 'particularly elusive' and there is a wide variation of educational standards and practice in the area. They hope the UK Confederation of Hypnotherapy Organisations will be a more successful initiative. And there are some doctors and dentists who practise hypnotherapy: many are members of the Society of Medical and Dental Hypnosis.

Massage therapies — Some massage treatments fall within the remit of beauty treatments but Mills and Budd only surveyed those that emphasise the health benefits of massage. They identified nine professional groups representing massage therapists and two umbrella organisations. The newest of these, the British Association for Massage Therapy, has been most successful at attracting the larger professional bodies and combines the four largest groups. However it is worth noting that many massage therapists also apply aromatherapy and may therefore be members of aromatherapy organisations or multidisciplinary organisations.

Naturopathy and nutrition — Although Mills and Budd looked at these two groups together they concluded they were different enough to justify the fact that they have different aspirations. The naturopaths are currently represented by two main voluntary bodies and the largest of these two bodies, the General Council and Register for Naturopaths, is actively moving to achieve consensus on regulation in the discipline. The nutritional therapists (non medical) are currently represented by three main groups although a new umbrella body, the Nutritional Therapy Council, has recently been set up to focus specifically on education and the development of National Occupational Standards. The largest of the nutritional therapy groups, the British Association of Nutritional Therapists, see a chance for the new Council to start playing a role in co-ordinating training colleges.

Reflexology — There are many groups representing reflexologists, but there have been attempts to achieve consensus among them over recent years, particularly towards agreeing National Occupational Standards for the discipline. As part of a wider project with the Department of Health Mills and Budd identified the reflexologists as a useful pilot group to explore the practicalities of achieving greater consensus within a discipline. One outcome of this exercise is the recent launch of the Reflexology Forum that aims to represent every reflexologist in the country.

Shiatsu — Shiatsu was the only therapy which Mills and Budd found had become more fragmented over the past three years, even though it was originally a well-organised profession under one professional body. Over the past two years two new Shiatsu bodies have been created, resulting in five bodies overall. The Shiatsu Society, the oldest and largest Shiatsu body, supports the idea of statutory regulation, while the other Shiatsu bodies disagree and believe Shiatsu should remain voluntarily regulated.

Source: Mills, S. & Budd, S. (2000) (Op.cit.).

5.8 It is clear from Box 2 that the nature of the voluntary regulatory structures varies considerably across the CAM professions. In the light of such variations we asked the Department of Health if they were concerned about the lack of statutory controls in this area. The Department of Health made it clear that within each profession "CAM practitioners and products are currently subject to a wide range of statutory and non-statutory controls. Any concerns that CAM is insufficiently regulated must be set out in the context of this wide range of measures" (P 101). They outlined areas, shown in Box 3, where CAM is already subject to regulation of a general nature.

Box 3

General Statutory Regulation of CAM

- The Health and Safety at Work etc. Act 1974 and its associated Regulations place a statutory duty on employers and the self-employed to ensure the health and safety of people affected by various activities undertaken on their premises;

- The Food Safety Act 1990 controls the sale and supply of non-medical products for human consumption, which includes some products associated with CAM;

- The provisions of the Trade Descriptions Act 1968 and the Consumer Protection Act 1987 are enforced by local authority Trading Standards Officers, and apply to professions which make claims for the goods or services they sell, including complementary therapists;

- There is legislation relating to specific illnesses and medical conditions — for example, cancer and venereal disease — which prohibits non-medically qualified individuals from purporting to cure, or in some cases treat, them;

- Many organisations which represent complementary therapists are registered charities or limited companies (or both) under the Charities and Companies Acts, and are subject to the provisions of those Acts;

- The London Local Authorities Act 1991 requires the licensing of premises used for activities which include acupuncture, massage, and other special treatments;

- Under common law all practitioners have a duty of care towards their patients;

- In the private sector there is a contractual relationship between therapist and client, which is legally enforceable.

Source: Department of Health (P 104).

5.9 Another factor to be taken into consideration in relation to the regulation of CAM is that of the legal requirements for the practice of medicine. The Common Law right to practise medicine means that in the United Kingdom anyone can treat a sick person even if they have no training in any type of healthcare whatsoever, provided that the individual treated has given informed consent. (Treatment without consent constitutes an assault.) Persons exercising this right must not identify themselves by any of the titles protected by statute and they cannot prescribe medicines that are regulated prescription-only drugs. This means that, as long as they do not claim to be a medical practitioner registered under the Medical Act, then anyone can offer medical advice and treatment and can purport to treat a range of diseases, provided that they do not claim to cure or treat certain specified diseases as proscribed by law. The Common Law right to practise springs from the fundamental principle that everyone can choose the form of healthcare that they require. Thus, although statutory regulation can award a therapy protection of title, it cannot stop anyone utilising the methods of that therapy under a slightly different name.

5.10 Issues arising from the different position of medically qualified persons who practise CAM will be considered as a separate issue in the last section of this chapter.

WEAKNESSES OF THE CURRENT SITUATION

5.11 As the outline of the current regulatory situation indicates, there is considerable variation in the levels of professionalisation within the CAM world. Even within some therapeutic disciplines there is considerable fragmentation, sometimes resulting in several bodies, each with different training and educational requirements, codes of practice and complaints procedures, representing therapists in the same field.

5.12 The General Osteopathic Council (GOsC) (now a statutory regulatory body) referred to the time when the osteopathic profession had been highly fragmented and explained that: "This situation, inevitably, gave rise to considerable public confusion amongst members of the public" (Q 412). They also explained that once they had overcome this problem and developed a single statutory self-regulatory body this gave "members of the public who hitherto may have been reluctant to consult an osteopath the confidence to do so" (p 102). The experience of the osteopathic profession shows the benefits for the public and ultimately the profession of having a well-organised and coherent regulatory structure. One serious problem of therapies represented by several professional bodies is that the disciplinary procedures of those bodies have little weight; if a practitioner is struck off one register, he, or she, can find another. Not all therapies have yet reached a stage where the public can find reputable, well-trained practitioners. The public cannot have full confidence in those therapies where there is considerable professional fragmentation. **We recommend that, in order to protect the public, professions with more than one regulatory body make a concerted effort to bring their various bodies together and to develop a clear professional structure.**

5.13 There are currently no specific measures that affect the practice of CAM by practitioners trained abroad. Without statutory controls it is impossible to enforce entry criteria for practice in the United Kingdom. A considerable proportion of unregulated healthcare is, in fact, provided for British subjects of other ethnic origins, by practitioners of their own culture. This practice has raised particular concerns when it involves the import and supply of traditional medicines from areas in the world where European Union level production standards do not apply. The MCA, in their submission with the Department of Health, confirmed that herbal imports from Asia, Africa and elsewhere gave them some concern (Q 40).

Features of an Effective Regulatory System

5.14 The primary benefit of effective regulation is that it protects the public. This is done through five main features which the BMA outlined: "To provide a code of conduct, a disciplinary procedure, and a complaints procedure; to provide minimum standards of training and to supervise training courses and accreditation; to understand and advertise areas of competence, including limits of competence within each therapy; to keep an up to date register of qualified practitioners; and to provide and publicise information on CAM" (P 46).

5.15 The Department of Health commissioned Budd and Mills at the University of Exeter to develop a regulatory information pack (referred to in 5.1). In this pack they outline the modern principles of professional self-regulation in the health field. These are principles all CAM bodies should aim to work towards when developing their professional structures and are outlined in Box 4. This pack is a useful resource for all CAM bodies.

Box 4

Modern Principles of Statutory Self-Regulation in the Health Field

Regulatory bodies:

- Are accountable to the public and Parliament for their actions and performance.

- Must set clearly expressed standards of the knowledge, skills, experience, attitudes and values necessary for continuing practice.

- Should demonstrate that their activities are conducted in an open and clear manner.

- Should concern themselves with the competence and conduct of practitioners at all stages in their careers.

- Should not delay in taking action to protect patients from serious adverse outcomes of care when such circumstances arise.

- Should demonstrate their objectivity in making assessments and forming judgements about performance.

- Should show that their procedures are free of racial and other forms of bias and discrimination.

- Should take proper account of the health service context when making interventions.

- If involved in education, should produce clearly stated standards for professional education and training by which the providers of education and training can be monitored and held to account.

- Should operate clear and independent disputes procedures.

- Should supply appropriate and valid information on their regulatory activities.

- Should demonstrate an ability to work across different regulatory boundaries to develop consistent standards.

- Should retain high public confidence and have sufficient lay involvement to make an effective contribution in their governance and operation.

- Should ensure that those being regulated understand what is expected of them and the role of the regulatory body in relation to their practice and wider health services.

- Should review and update standards regularly taking account of feedback from patients, practitioners and other interested parties.

- Should ensure that their procedures are well-defined and transparent, that they are operated in a way that is fair and sensitive, and that their efforts to enforce standards are targeted in a way that is proportionate to the seriousness of the problems involved.

- Should work in partnership with the NHS and with other organisations that provide or manage healthcare, thus enabling NHS organisations to achieve high standards of quality care for all those for whom the NHS is responsible.

Source: Budd, S. & Mills, S. (2000) (Op.cit.).

Regulatory Options

VOLUNTARY SELF-REGULATION

5.16 The regulatory information pack produced by Budd and Mills outlined the features of a good voluntary self-regulatory body. These are also set out in Box 5.

5.17 There was general consensus among our witnesses that a good voluntary regulatory structure is needed for each CAM therapy before statutory regulation would be further considered. However, voluntary self-regulation, when administered by a single, professional body, is often thought to be enough to protect the patients and organise the practitioners of some therapies. We have heard a substantial amount of evidence suggesting that, in many circumstances, voluntary self-regulation may, when administered by a single professional body, be as effective as statutory regulation. Mr Michael McIntyre, speaking as a trustee of FIM, in response to a question, observed: "I think your point about it not being absolutely necessary to have statutory state regulation for risk of harm to be reduced, or to be monitored, is a good one. Provided the profession has all the self-regulatory mechanisms in place, there is no reason why it should do harm" (QQ 104 & 105).

Box 5

Features of an Effective Voluntary Self-Regulatory Body

An effective voluntary self-regulating professional body:

— maintains a register of individual members or member organisations;

— sets educational standards and runs an accreditation system for training establishments;

— maintains professional competence among its members with an adequate programme of Continuing Professional Development;

— provides codes of conduct, ethics and practice;

— has in place a complaints mechanism for members of the public;

— has in place a disciplinary procedure that is accessible to the public;

— requires members to have adequate professional indemnity insurance;

— has the capacity to represent the whole profession;

— includes external representation on executive councils to represent patients or clients and the wider public interest.

Source: Budd, S. & Mills, S. (2000) *(Op.cit.)*.

5.18 Some of the evidence we have received has made the point that, on the other hand, statutory regulation does offer greater power of control than voluntary regulation. Mr Michael McIntyre qualified his praise of good voluntary regulation with the point that "...there are certain benefits accruing out of statutory self-regulation for some professions which would not come otherwise." These would include, for example, prescription of certain restricted herbs and protection of title (QQ 104 & 105). Protection of title is particularly important, as it ensures that practitioners who have been struck off a register for misconduct cannot continue to practise under the title of a particular therapy.

5.19 Ms Julie Stone has written and lectured extensively on the subject of the regulation of CAM therapies. She provided evidence against the need for further statutory regulation of any CAM therapy. She suggested that statutory regulation was not needed to minimise risk to the public: "Whilst such risks as do exist are a matter of concern, the therapies which are most likely to give rise to harm are already the most effectively regulated, either by statute (in the case of osteopathy and chiropractic) or by effective voluntary self-regulation mechanisms (in the cases of acupuncture, homeopathy and herbalism). The only reason for expecting the statutory regulation of herbalists is because of the anomalies in the Medicines Act 1968 which currently permit unregulated practitioners to supply the public with potentially harmful medicinal products" (PP 286 & 287).

5.20 Ms Stone also argued that many of the risks of CAM are not inherent, but only exist if practitioners are not properly trained, and that a good voluntary self-regulatory structure could ensure practitioners were properly trained: "It is also important to separate the risks which are inherent in the therapy from risks which are far more likely to materialise if the practitioners are insufficiently trained...ensuring that practitioners are properly trained is certainly one aspect of effective regulation. The vital question is whether statutory regulation is the only way in which high standards can be assured. My opinion is that it is not" (P 287). She went on to cite the work of the British Acupuncture Accreditation Board as an example of the high standards which can be achieved within a voluntary self- regulatory context, adding that public awareness of voluntary regulatory bodies was important in order to marginalise practitioners outside such schemes (P 287).

5.21 Where there is no lead professional body, and where the various associations representing the therapy are disparate in the views that they hold regarding educational and training standards, there is a problem. We have, for example, been disturbed to read in evidence from the British Complementary Medicine Association (p 145) that some organisations are offering home study training courses which, on the basis of advertising material, seem seriously inadequate. In a situation where a therapy is represented by various disparate professional bodies it is very hard for the public to know where to look to find a 'competent' therapist. Therefore the voluntary regulatory system might be inadequate. Ms Julie Stone acknowledged this but suggested there would be less merit in forcing statutory regulation on such therapies than there would be in aiding the development of a better voluntary regulatory structure: "I would support any moves which encourage the development of a single professional register for each therapy, although I would challenge whether this should imply a move towards statutory regulation for therapies where the risk of harm to the public is less acute. There are various ways in which the Government could support such initiatives, including introducing education and training grants and/or fees for those studying on an accredited professional course (as is the case in medicine and nursing)" (P 287).

5.22 Ms Julie Stone concluded her evidence by saying: "The current professionalisation taking place within CAM is to be encouraged. Effective voluntary regulation and the existence of single professional registers can provide many of the safeguards of statutory regulation. Voluntary self-regulation is less expensive to administer and for that reason alone carries the support of many practitioners. Since incidence of serious harm appears to be low, and is equally capable of arising in a statutory context, there would seem to be no justification at the present time for introducing mandatory licensing or statutory regulation for all practitioners. Nonetheless, there may be an argument for requiring, as a minimum safety precaution, that all practitioners carry professional indemnity insurance, so that a patient who sues a practitioner can seek damages through the courts" (P 287).

5.23 For the therapies in our Groups 2 and 3 we are in agreement with Julie Stone's argument. A good voluntary regulatory structure is needed before a profession can seek statutory regulatory status. None of the therapies in Groups 2 and 3 has yet united under one professional body, and so statutory regulation is not a viable option for them at the present time. Indeed, for the disciplines we have listed in Group 3, such a prospect seems to us remote. For therapies in Group 2 the inherent risks of the therapies are minimal, and most are used as a complement to conventional medicine and not as an alternative, but to ensure that the public are protected from rogue practitioners, and have clear reliable information on these therapies, a good voluntary regulatory structure would be of benefit. **Therefore, we recommend that practitioners of each of the therapies in Group 2 should organise themselves under a single professional body for each therapy. These bodies should be well-promoted so that the public who access these therapies are aware of them. Each should comply with core professional principles, and relevant information about each body should be made known to medical practitioners and other healthcare professionals. Patients could then have a single, reliable point of reference for standards, and would be protected against the risk of poorly-trained practitioners and have redress for poor service.**

STATUTORY REGULATION

5.24 Statutory regulation has the same aims and functions as good quality voluntary regulation; the desirable features of statutory regulation are therefore very similar to those achieved under voluntary self-regulation. The difference is that statutory regulation has the force of the law to ensure that its aims are met.

5.25 There are three routes to achieving statutory regulation. The first is for a profession or therapy to pursue its own Act of Parliament which establishes a statutory regulating body. The second and third are to pursue statutory regulation through the provisions of the Health Act 1999, which provides two separate options for achieving statutory regulation. Option one allows new regulatory bodies to be set up by order, subject to affirmative resolution in both Houses of Parliament. Option two allows professions to take advantage of the new Health Professions Council which will replace the Council for Professions Supplementary to Medicine. The Health Act allows new professions to join the previously closed group of professions within the Council. (These routes are reviewed below).

5.26 There are several advantages of statutory regulation, all of which derive from the legal backing afforded and the respect of the rest of the healthcare professions, which derive from having achieved statutory recognition. The advantage most often articulated to us was protection of title, so that only practitioners who are registered with the relevant statutory regulatory body can legally use a particular title. This provision makes it very easy for the public to determine who is, and who is not, a properly qualified practitioner, and gives the relevant professional body the power to determine who can claim to practise the therapy in question. The Consumers' Association explained the importance of this: "...unless you have protection of title you have little control over the practitioner who has no training, or has training and has been taken off the register" (Q 841).

5.27 The second main advantage of statutory regulation is the legal establishment of a single register of practitioners. This makes it easy for the public to find out who is, and who is not, qualified and trained properly and also makes tracking of practitioners easier. This could be done by voluntary regulatory bodies which provide a register of practitioners, but without protection of title there is little opportunity to ensure that those not on the register do not mislead the public into thinking they are adequately qualified and trained therapists. The Consumers' Association also articulated the importance of the public having a single reference point that covers all practitioners in a field, saying: "Consumers should be able to contact a body to establish if the practitioner they are going to see is indeed registered" (Q 840).

5.28 The third advantage of statutory regulation is the legal underpinning of a body's disciplinary procedures so that a practitioner struck off a list due to misconduct has nowhere else to register and can no longer use the title the list had bestowed upon him.

5.29 All these features could probably be achieved by well-publicised voluntary regulation. However, for therapies with high inherent risk it is probably desirable to have legal underpinning of these provisions.

5.30 FIM added another advantage of statutory regulation to this list. Mr Michael McIntyre, a Trustee of FIM, told us: "...there are certain benefits accruing out of statutory self-regulation for some professions which would not come otherwise. For example, there may be actual medicines...which the regulatory authorities would not want on the market generally and those would only be available to those who were actually in some way state registered, as doctors are" (Q 104).

5.31 However, one of the main advantages of statutory regulation, protection of title, is not as clear-cut as it may seem. Although statutory regulation does provide protection of title, the common law right to practise medicine means that anyone can use the techniques of a therapy, even if it is statutory regulated, as long as they do not identify themselves by using the title which is protected. The GOsC explained that there is "...a difference between a restriction of title and a functional closure. We have, under the Osteopaths Act, a protection of title only, so it is possible for members of the medical profession or physiotherapists to use osteopathic techniques provided they do not hold themselves to be an osteopathic practitioner...it was felt at the time of the Act going through Parliament that it would be inappropriate and, indeed, impossible to produce a functional closure" (QQ 421 & 422). We have learned that some former osteopathic practitioners, refused registration under the Act, continue to practise, for example, as osteomyologists or cranio-sacral practitioners.

5.32 There are also some disadvantages to statutory regulation. These come in two forms: difficulties that arise from the process of achieving statutory regulation; and the potential effects of statutory regulation itself. The main concern about the effects of regulation is that regulation of a therapy may restrict consumer choice. Statutory regulation is expensive to set up and its very nature restricts the number of practitioners. If a therapy does not have appropriate numbers of therapists and resources for statutory regulation then the process may cause the professional bodies to lose money and make it impossible for some individuals to register as practitioners. The Consumers' Association explained that: "To over-regulate may make particular therapies inaccessible to people, and we do not feel that would be appropriate either" (Q 832). The British Complementary Medicine Association also articulated this view, stating: "perhaps to use statutory regulation for complementary therapies is like using a sledge hammer to crack a nut" (Q 610).

5.33 However, the idea that statutory regulation may restrict consumer choice is not necessarily true. Statutory regulation could even have the opposite effect by giving consumers the confidence to consult practitioners whom they might not otherwise consult due to concerns about regulation. And it is not necessarily true that statutory regulation, by its very nature, restricts the number of practitioners of a therapy. It is true that, in the short term, statutory regulation might prevent a few practitioners from using a particular professional title on the basis that they were not judged to be sufficiently well qualified or competent. In the medium term, a profession regulated by statute is far more likely to attract students to its accredited colleges, partly because career advisers are much more likely to recommend such professions to their students.

ROUTES TO STATUTORY REGULATION

Own Act

5.34 Until the provisions of the Health Act 1999 came into force, healthcare professions seeking statutory regulation have had to seek it through primary legislation (except for the Professions Supplementary to Medicine).

5.35 The two CAM professions that have followed this route are the osteopaths, who achieved statutory recognition through the Osteopaths Act 1993, and the chiropractors who achieved statutory recognition through the Chiropractors Act 1994[38]. The features of the GOsC and the GCC, which were set up under the two Acts, can be seen in Appendix 2.

5.36 We talked to both the GOsC and the GCC about their experience of statutory regulation.

---

[38] Both Acts were taken through the House of Lords by Lord Walton of Detchant, who chaired the Sub-Committee which prepared this Report.

5.37 The GOsC told us that they could not think of any disadvantages, from the patients' perspective, of statutory regulation (Q 465). They did say that from the profession's point of view some would argue that the process of achieving statutory regulation has been "complicated and difficult" (Q 465). However, they qualified this statement by saying: "In the final analysis the profession will be stronger and patients will benefit more from the process" (Q 465). The GOsC explained that the cost in terms of what each practitioner has to pay each year is similar to what most of them were paying under the voluntary system (Q 466). However, they did raise a note of caution for smaller therapies which may not have as many practitioners to spread the costs: "...there is a certain limit, a certain sum of money, which a statutory body...does require...and therefore, professions which are small in number would have to think very seriously about whether they could actually afford to have a system of statutory regulation in place" (Q 466). The GOsC stated that the cost per annum of their body is likely to reach £1.8 million, with at present about 2,000 registered osteopaths.

5.38 The GCC were more outspoken about the problems they had faced in achieving their Act. Mrs Norma Morris, Chairman of the GCC, told us that it is "...a very onerous system" (Q 470). She added: "...I doubt whether it would be suitable for all the professions that may seek that status. I hope that it would be possible to find some sort of half way house for such practitioners...One problem is that despite the very best intentions of all the civil servants with whom we have worked, there is a difficulty in getting business done through the Department of Health...and also there is the question of start-up funds for new bodies" (Q 470). However she did say that statutory regulation was "a very desirable system and one that has benefits for the public" (Q 470). It is clearly important that the Department of Health should deploy sufficient staff and resources to deal with future regulatory applications.

5.39 Each Act has tended to make provisions which could in the past only be amended through primary legislation which can take a very long time. With the passage of the Health Act, amendments can be made by Order in Council.

5.40 Neither the GOsC nor the GCC highlighted any problems with the status of being regulated by statute. They felt it increased public safety and public confidence, as well as professional respect and the standard of organisation within the profession itself. The negative feelings they did articulate were all concerned with the time, cost and complications of the process of getting their Act drafted and through Parliament. The Health Act provides for the same level of statutory regulation, but through a less onerous system (discussed below). Therefore the process of achieving an individual professional Act is no longer necessary, but the advantages of statutory regulation remain, and the lessons learnt by the GOsC and the GCC will be very valuable to other professions. It is also worth noting that many of the problems experienced by the osteopaths arose from the fact that they were setting up from scratch, with no State funding, a new and innovative statutory regulatory mechanism, with no precedent in healthcare legislation for the previous 40 years. Professions in the future seeking statutory regulation will have a wealth of knowledge and experience upon which to draw.

Health Act 1999

5.41 The Health Act 1999 provides two main opportunities for healthcare professions aspiring to achieve statutory regulation; the first of these is the opportunity for a single body representing the entire profession to apply for statutory regulation by Order in the Privy Council, in contrast to pursuing its own Act of Parliament. The second opportunity is by virtue of the abolition of the Council of Professions Supplementary to Medicine (CPSM) which is being replaced by the Health Professions Council, furnished with new provisions and wider powers.

5.42 In their evidence the Department of Health said that they envisaged the provisions laid out in the Health Act as being advantageous to professions with a good voluntary structure: "To help all healthcare professionals improve the current levels of self-regulation, the Government took powers in the Health Act 1999 to enable existing professions to modernise their legislative provisions and to provide a statutory self-regulatory framework for those professions whose members supported such a system" (P 106). With specific reference to the opportunities afforded to CAM bodies by the Health Act, FIM referred to a speech by Tessa Jowell MP, the then Minister for Health, who told them in May 1999 how it would be possible for aspiring CAM professions to attain statutory self-regulation using the provisions of the Health Act, provided they met certain conditions. The Department of Health made it clear to us that they saw the Health Act 1999 as being advantageous, in that it will "enable existing statutory schemes to be strengthened and statutory schemes for other professions to be introduced" (Q 5).

5.43 The Department of Health are not yet clear as to how the practicalities of the Health Act will work. Yvette Cooper MP, Parliamentary Under Secretary of State for Public Health, said she was unable, as yet, to clarify the advantages and disadvantages of each route to regulation offered by the

Act, nor how it would be decided which route a therapy should take. When we asked her what advantages a therapy would gain from coming under the Health Professions Council, as opposed to achieving statutory status in its own right, she told us: "I think it is probably too early to give a definite answer to that question. There is clearly, in all these regulatory issues, a trade-off between, on the one hand, having an individual regulatory organisation for individual professions that have sufficient expertise to regulate themselves…and, at the same time, having critical mass within the organisations and having proper co-ordination between them where regulatory issues are in common or overlap…I think we do not have closed minds on this at all" (Q 1876). Professor Liam Donaldson, Chief Medical Officer, told us that the Department of Health have recently published a consultation document on the Health Professions Council and are awaiting responses on that (due in early November) before moving ahead (Q 1876). Despite these uncertainties there is a generally positive view amongst the CAM world towards the provisions of the Health Act.

5.44 FIM sees the Health Act as lifting some of the burden which therapies previously faced when pursuing their own Act: "…the NHS Bill…now gives much greater flexibility in terms of approaching statutory self-regulation. The path which the chiropractors and osteopaths had to go down was through a Private Member's Bill, which was terribly long and drawn out and does not give the sort of flexibility which the new arrangements potentially do" (Q 102). Yvette Cooper MP expanded on the flexibility of the Health Act: "I think that the Health Act provides several advantages in that it allows us to become more responsive to the needs of the health profession and to the Health Service. That has been a problem with the previous situation where any amendment or changes, whether it be new professions coming aboard or changes in the nature of the profession…requires primary legislation that has been a very cumbersome and slow process and has resulted, over a long period of time, in changes that might otherwise have happened not being able to take place for that reason. I think that the Health Act provides advantages in terms of responsiveness. Where there is widespread support, and a proper consultation has been gone through, I think it would allow us to put an effective statutory regulation framework in place much more smoothly and rapidly than we might otherwise be able to do" (Q 1878).

5.45 The GOsC, which has had the experience of the single Act route, also thought that the provisions of the Health Act offered a good opportunity for other CAM professions. "Recent changes in the powers given to the Secretary of State and proposed legislation to supersede the current Professions Supplementary to Medicine Act 1960 could help to facilitate the process of statutory regulation for some of the professions which have reached the appropriate stage of development" (p 102). Mr Simon Fielding, Chairman of the GOsC, elaborated: "I think those provisions [envisaged under the Health Act] do offer a very useful method for complementary medical practitioners and groups to consider, and certainly would obviate the need for going for a single parliamentary Bill…So in a sense, those provisions certainly facilitate those professions that are ready to make that transition" (Q 414).

5.46 To understand the option of coming under the Health Professions Council, provided by the Health Act, it is necessary to understand the old CPSM. The Council was set up under the Professions Supplementary to Medicine Act 1960 and has supervised the activity of specialist boards representing twelve professions: art, music and drama therapy; chiropody; clinical scientists in health; dietetics; medical laboratory science; occupational therapy; orthoptics; paramedics; physiotherapy; prosthetics and orthotics; radiography; and speech and language therapists. Each of the boards maintained a register of practitioners, had a role in regulating and overseeing training which led to State registration, and also sifted applications for state registration and cancelled registration in cases of misconduct. The Council's role was that it financed each of the boards, arranged and monitored elections for each board's membership and supervised and co-ordinated each board's work. However there were deficiencies in the Council's ability to monitor practitioners as it was not illegal for an unregistered practitioner to use the title of one of the professions in the Council for Professions Supplementary to Medicine's remit as long as the term 'state registered' was not used[39].

5.47 Another limitation of the Council was that it could not register any further groups as they have reached the limit of twelve professional boards set out in the Professions Supplementary to Medicine Act 1960 (P 72).

5.48 Clause 47 of the Health Act 1999 addresses the problems faced by the CPSM by replacing it with a new regulatory body called the Health Professions Council. The main differences between the new Health Professions Council and the CPSM are as follows:

---

[39] Budd, S. & Mills, S. (2000) *(Op.cit.)*.

- Protection of title: this will mean that no-one can use the title of any of the professions within the Council's remit unless they are on the Council's register. This should remove public confusion and increase public protection.

- Increased accountability: there will be new disciplinary powers which will include reprimands, suspension pending retraining, and fines.

- A new health committee: to deal with registrants who put the public at risk because they themselves are ill, with the power to suspend registration until registrants have recovered.

- Lay representation: and a shift of power from the CPSM's boards to a central council.

5.49 The Health Professions Council will also have the ability to register new groups (P 72). The provisions which a profession will need to meet to be eligible to come under the new Health Professions Council will be the same as the criteria were to join the CPSM and are reviewed in Box 6 below. Any CAM profession wishing to come under the Health Professions Council will need to meet these criteria.

Box 6

Criteria for Petitioning to come under the Council for Professions Supplementary to Medicine or its Successor

1. Is there a need for the public to be protected from the activities of the group in that their work involves invasive procedures or clinical intervention with the potential for harm or can the exercise of judgement by the unsupervised professional significantly impact on patient health or welfare where such procedures or judgement are not already regulated by other means such as through supervision or other legislation?

2. Does the group naturally fall within the family of health professions and conventional medicine?

3. Can the group be considered to be a mature profession? The nine definitions given by the late Lord Benson in a House of Lords debate on 8 July 1992 are used as a general test (see Box 7).

4. Has the group a single, defined professional voice which can speak for it and does it work to a common level of threshold competency?

5. Is there a common education system at an appropriate level which would allow a unified approach to the approval of course programmes and the establishments providing them?

6. Is the group large enough to provide the additional body of unpaid volunteers to fill the necessary offices at the CPSM or its successor in turn and to undertake the considerable work inherent in the statutory regulation of a profession?

7. Can the group statutorily fall within the Professions Supplementary to Medicine Act or its successor? This is a requirement as it could, on investigation, be found that the activities of a group could partly fall within or significantly impinge upon a group or groups being regulated under other Acts.

Source: Council for Professions Supplementary to Medicine.

Box 7

Criteria for a Group to be Considered a Profession

1. The profession must be controlled by a governing body which in professional matters directs the behaviour of its members. For their part the members have a responsibility to subordinate their selfish private interests in favour of support for the governing body.

2. The governing body must set adequate standards of education as a condition of entry and thereafter ensure that students obtain an acceptable standard of professional competence. Training and education do not stop at qualification. They must continue throughout the member's professional life.

3. The governing body must set the ethical rules and professional standards which are to be observed by the members. They should be higher than those established by the general law.

4. The rules and standards enforced by the governing body should be designed for the benefit of the public and not for the private advantage of the members.

5. The governing body must take disciplinary action including, if necessary, expulsion from membership should the rules and standards it lays down not be observed or should a member be guilty of bad professional work.

6. Work is often reserved to a profession by statute – not for the advantage of the members but because, for the protection of the public, it should be carried out only by persons with the requisite training, standards and disciplines.

7. The governing body must satisfy itself that there is fair and open competition in the practice of the profession so that the public are not at risk of being exploited. It follows that members in practice must give information to the public about their experience, competence, capacity to do the work and the fees payable.

8. The members of the profession, whether in practice or in employment, must be independent in thought and outlook. They must be willing to speak their minds without fear or favour. They must not allow themselves to be put under the control or dominance of any person or organisation which could impair that independence.

9. In its specific field of learning a profession must give leadership to the public it serves.

Source: Council for Professions Supplementary to Medicine.

5.50 The provisions of the Health Act are a step forward in easing the path of health professions that wish to achieve statutory status. How much easier this route will be remains to be seen. Our discussions with the Department of Health indicate some uncertainty over how they will decide which route, under the Health Act, a therapy should follow to achieve statutory status, even though it will be the Department of Health itself that will decide which route is most appropriate for each therapy, after discussion with that body. We believe there are some therapies that would benefit from statutory regulation and should use the opportunities provided by the Health Act. These are reviewed below.

WHICH THERAPIES WOULD BENEFIT FROM STATUTORY REGULATION?

5.51 The Department of Health's written evidence stated that the Government does not see a need to single out additional CAM professions for special regulation. However they go on to say: "There is scope for the larger professions to follow the osteopaths and chiropractors in gaining statutory self-regulation, and this would undoubtedly serve their professions well. However there are also ways in which other professions could strengthen their self-regulation without statutory powers. For them the first step must be the formation of a lead self-regulatory body for each profession" (P 101).

5.52 However we are aware that since submitting their written evidence in December 1999 the Government have now identified acupuncture and herbal medicine as specific therapies they would like to see achieve statutory regulation. This was something that Yvette Cooper MP, Parliamentary Under Secretary of State for Public Health, told us at the end of our Inquiry: "I think we would support their moves towards statutory regulation…We would strongly encourage them to continue the process towards proper self-regulation and statutory regulation as well…We do think that in the area of acupuncture and herbal medicine it is perhaps more important than in other areas. Whilst we have done considerable work, particularly with Exeter University, in providing support and detailed information for all professions in terms of increasing self-regulation, for these two we think we need to take additional steps. One of the issues we are looking at, at the moment, is whether or not we should be setting a timetable for moves towards statutory regulation, and we are considering producing a consultation paper on that at the moment" (Q 1875). We welcome this approach.

5.53 The Osteopathic and Chiropractic professions are now regulated by law. **It is our opinion that acupuncture and herbal medicine are the two therapies which are at a stage where it would be of benefit to them and their patients if the practitioners strive for statutory regulation under the Health Act 1999, and we recommend that they should do so. Statutory regulation may also be appropriate eventually for the non-medical homeopaths.**

5.54 Our main criterion for determining the need for statutory regulation is whether the therapy poses significant risk to the public from its practice. We believe that both acupuncture and herbal medicine do carry inherent risk, beyond the extrinsic risk that all CAMs pose, which is the risk of omission of conventional medical treatment. Our other criteria for determining the desirability of statutory regulation include whether the therapy in question has a sufficiently well organised voluntary regulatory system, and a consensus among its members that statutory regulation is the desired next step for the profession. Although if a therapy posed significant intrinsic risks and had a poor voluntary regulatory structure, it might be worth the Department of Health putting pressure on that therapy to come under a statutory regulatory system, we were not made aware of any such cases. A final consideration in determining the desirability of statutory regulation is whether the therapy in question has a credible evidence base to support its claims. As statutory regulation is likely to increase the profile of a therapy it is important that there is evidence of benefit to patients suffering from the conditions it purports to treat as well as evidence that it carries few adverse effects.

5.55 If the professions of acupuncture and herbal medicine receive statutory regulatory status, then all but one of the therapies in our Group 1 will have statutory status. The present position with respect to homeopathy is less clear-cut. Medical practitioners who are members of the Faculty of Homeopathy are already regulated by the General Medical Council (GMC). The Faculty wish to see introduced a form of regulation of the non-medical homeopaths who are less certain of the potential advantages. We do not at present make any formal recommendation about the homeopathic profession but, nevertheless, feel that statutory regulation may ultimately be appropriate. **Other professions must strive to come together under one voluntary self-regulating body with the appropriate features outlined in Box 5, and some may wish ultimately to aim to move towards regulation under the Health Act once they are unified with a single voice.**

5.56 We heard evidence from the principal professional associations associated with acupuncture and herbal medicine to canvass their opinions on obtaining statutory regulatory status. We also talked to the Homeopathic associations about their views on this subject:

Acupuncture

5.57 In the case of acupuncture we heard from the British Acupuncture Council, the largest body representing non-statutory registered acupuncturists. They told us that they were well prepared to take the next step towards statutory regulation: "…we have been on a long path of voluntary self-regulation over the last 20 years. We now have a single umbrella body with the British Acupuncture Council. We have the educational standards, codes of practice, of ethics, and of professional conduct, which we can enforce. We have taken many steps along the road on a voluntary basis" (Q 769).

5.58 However, the British Acupuncture Council also told us that they had not yet reached consensus on whether they should take the step towards statutory regulation: "… initial debates within our community of acupuncturists have shown that opinion is somewhat divided on this point. There are concerns by some of our members around loss of autonomy and the cost involved in statutory self-regulation. However, on an informal basis, the profession is leading towards exploring the issues of regulation in more depth. We formed, for example, a Regulation Action Group, with expert advisers joining us, to look at the issues in more depth. We are starting patient focus groups to look at the patient perspective, and what would be in the interests of patients in terms of any moves towards statutory regulation: and informal discussion with osteopaths, to find out what we can learn from the path they have taken. As has been mentioned, we have made informal approaches to the Department of Health…but we would stress we need to carry the membership in any decision that we would move towards in terms of statutory self-regulation" (Q 769).

5.59 This evidence shows that under the guidance of the British Acupuncture Council the acupuncturists have worked hard to establish a voluntary regulatory structure which is commendable. They now have the prerequisites to obtain statutory regulatory status. Their concerns over taking this next step are founded on the ability to obtain a unanimous membership decision because their members may fear a reduction in their autonomy and an increase in the costs for which they are liable. We hope that these two fears will not prohibit this large, well-organised profession from striving to obtain statutory regulatory status. As we have discussed previously, the cost of achieving statutory regulation has been reduced with the provisions of the Health Act. The acupuncturists should also bear in mind the increased public and cross-professional confidence likely to result from statutory status; this will, we hope, allay their fears.

Herbal Medicine

5.60 The European Herbal Practitioners Association, who represent the majority of United Kingdom herbalists, told us: "We feel that our future holds, in terms of statutory self-regulation, mostly prospects and benefits: the benefits for our members, but equally benefits to all the public, in ensuring competencies and safe practice. We do not see any threats. We do see uncertainties, however. There is still uncertainty about precisely what the 1999 Health Act will entail. It is a slightly different process to the one followed by osteopaths and chiropractors, so there is a certain amount that is unknown in regards to cost and financial implications"(Q 727). When asked if they thought the majority of medical herbalists will wish to seek statutory self-regulation they responded by saying yes, they did. The major incentive for this would be that there are a number of potentially harmful herbal medicines which they wish to be able to use, and currently are able to use under a schedule attached to the Medicines Act 1968. They expect that should they achieve statutory self-regulation, then registered professional herbal practitioners would be able to continue using those herbs (Q 728). The regulation of herbal practitioners is of course a separate issue from the regulation of herbal medicinal products. However the complicated issue of the status of herbal medicinal products will be discussed separately in the last section of this chapter.

Homeopathy

5.61 The non–medical homeopaths were much the least enthusiastic of the three therapies in our Group 1 about pursuing statutory status. The Society of Homoeopaths told us: "I think it is true to say that we have decided that voluntary self-regulation is our current option but I would like to emphasise that we have also used the qualifying phrase "for the time being" because there are two strands to that if you like. One is to observe very closely and monitor the progress and experience of the osteopaths and chiropractors in their role post-statutory self-regulation. We do realise it has not been quite as seamless as it might have been in that perhaps there are building blocks, foundations, to regulation that were not necessarily in place before the statute was passed. So, for the Society we have recognised that we need to develop a very strong self-regulating profession with those key building blocks in place and then examine whether or not regulation by statute is appropriate (Q 687). "We look at it as an open question. We realise that the issue of protection of title is a very important one but currently we are not sure that it has been fully addressed by statutory regulation in that, as has already been said this morning, it is recognised that as soon as you make laws there are ways around it" (Q 688).

5.62 However the Faculty of Homeopathy, representing the medical homeopaths, already regulated by the GMC, told us: "We do strongly believe that to be the case [that homeopathy should only be practised by those statutorily registered]. This does not mean that the current practitioners who do good homeopathic work in the community should not continue to do so but perhaps their kind of practice should be regulated in such a way that it falls within safe practice. It perhaps calls for a new sort of profession of homeopathic practitioner" (Q 651).

5.63 Of all the professions in our Group 1, homeopathy carries the fewest inherent risks in its practice, at least in relation to the consumption of homeopathic medicines. We are also aware that there is unusually strong contention about the evidence available for its efficacy. These two points could be seen as arguments against statutory regulation which could be considered unnecessary due to the limited risks and could also be seen as awarding a degree of legitimacy to a therapy about which much of the conventional scientific world has strong doubts and reservations. However, in our opinion there are reasons why homeopathy should still consider progressing towards statutory regulation. While the practice of homeopathy may itself be free from risk, it does create an opportunity for diverting conventional diagnosis and treatment away from patients with conditions where conventional treatment is well-established, as some patients seem to see it as offering a complete alternative to conventional medicine. Such attitudes mean that homeopaths are in a position of great responsibility. It is imperative that there is a way of ensuring that this position is handled professionally, that all homeopaths are registered, that they know the limits of their competence, and that there are disciplinary procedures with real teeth in place. Protection of title and a single statutory register would help ensure that this happens. It would also be encouraging if there was more collaboration between the medical homeopaths of the Faculty and the non-medical homeopaths of the Society, with more communication and agreement over information services for the public, making their options in choosing a homeopath clear, and with agreed educational standards to ensure that all those practising homeopathy are trained in homeopathic practice to a similar level. If the Society had statutory status, it might well facilitate communication and collaboration between them and the Faculty (see paras 5.84 – 5.86). Under the Society of Homoeopaths, the non-medical homeopaths have organised themselves well and their professional organisation should mean the transition to statutory regulation does not present too great an upheaval. For these reasons we would urge them eventually to consider the benefits they may derive from statutory regulation.

SINGLE UMBRELLA REGULATORY BODY?

5.64 We have also considered the option of a single "umbrella" regulatory body to cover all CAM therapies, or a significant number of them. There are currently several umbrella CAM voluntary regulatory bodies which plan to regulate practitioners from a range of different disciplines

5.65 We received written evidence from the Institute for Complementary Medicine, one such umbrella body. They told us: "The Institute for Complementary Medicine favours a single Act which recognises the autonomous divisions of specialist treatments as being the most beneficial, cost effective and efficient method of protecting professional practitioners whilst offering a transparent service to the public" (P 136). However, we are uncertain as to what they would do to overcome the fact that the diverse range of therapies which come under the title of CAM have a huge range of different educational and regulatory needs, while some have a weak, or even non-existent, evidence base[40].

5.66 We also heard from the British Complementary Medicine Association. This claims to be "…the major Complementary Medicine multi-therapy umbrella body in the United Kingdom, representing some 45 single therapy organisations (some of which are in themselves umbrella bodies for a single therapy)" (P 32). The British Complementary Medicine Association told us how they thought the diversities could be overcome so that therapies could unite under one body: "The first breakdown should be into alternative and complementary, as we have defined it. That gives you a good structure - those who make a medical diagnosis and those who do not. Then you come to the others. The system we operate is that each therapy has its own organisation and some of them have achieved an umbrella group for themselves in one therapy. What we would like to do is to say that a therapy must get together, whether it is inside the British Complementary Medicine Association or not. There is only one way to go, which is to get a body representing all the therapists in a particular therapy. That is the way, we feel, that you can combine strength, good practice, good regulation and so on" (Q 622).

5.67 The option of a single umbrella body was not favoured by most of the evidence we received, including the evidence of the Department of Health. Yvette Cooper MP, Parliamentary Under Secretary of State for Public Health, told us that she "would be personally uneasy about going too rapidly towards umbrella organisations that do not have sufficient concentrated expertise or thoroughness when it comes to regulating a particular area" (Q 1876). We recommend against it for several reasons. Umbrella groups do not, in themselves, obviate the need for all practitioners within one particular discipline to come together and agree standards of training, professional practice and requirements for Continuing Professional Development. It is impossible adequately to enforce any code of practice unless these basic fundamental provisions are in place. In short, common codes of practice are irrelevant until there are agreed standards of clinical care for each discipline and only the practitioners of each discipline can determine this by coming together and achieving a consensus. Umbrella bodies may also give a cloak of respectability to practitioners who may have minimal training in one or more of the different therapies. They may also encourage multi-therapy practitioners who want to mix a number of different therapies without being properly trained in one or more of them. There is an argument that anyone practising more than one therapy should at least have a grounding in a discrete clinical discipline so they have been exposed to training in basic medical sciences.

Regulation of Conventional Healthcare Professionals Practising CAM

5.68 The current position relating to the regulation of statutory regulated health professionals such as doctors, nurses, dentists and veterinary surgeons, who wish to incorporate CAM practice into their repertoire of therapies is very different from the position of CAM practitioners.

5.69 The GMC, the regulatory body for doctors, gave evidence to us. The code of ethics and disciplinary procedures of the GMC extend to the use of all the therapies a doctor may use in treating patients and therefore the GMC is responsible for regulating the use of all CAM therapies by doctors. They acknowledged that under the Medical Act 1983 a registered medical practitioner is technically

---

[40] Although the GMC represents doctors from a diverse range of specialties, a single regulatory body is appropriate as they all have the same basic training and core of knowledge, a claim which cannot be made for all CAM therapies.

free to practise any form of CAM or other therapy they believe will help their patients (Q 1045). However, they told us that "...we would wish them to practise within their competence. If they practised outwith their competence we would have strong views on that" (Q 1045). "These individuals need to be appropriately trained for the practice that they are going to be pursuing. So there is a gradation of training from undergraduate to post-graduate and then when problems do arise there is the policeman role of the General Medical Council, which will deal with a very small minority of medical practitioners. It is an unfortunate necessity" (Q 1061).

5.70 The GMC acknowledged that problems may arise with doctors practising CAM poorly and needing to be subject to a disciplinary action that might be consistent with a CAM regulatory body's process, but inconsistent with a GMC disciplinary process. Because of this they stated that "...it does mean that where such a body could be set up the interaction with the General Medical Council has got to be very close...there is no reason to doubt that there could be a very smooth interaction between such regulatory bodies. The example, I think, is again the General Dental Council and the General Medical Council, which has worked extremely well" (Q 1051).

5.71 The GMC also explained that they could discipline a doctor, not only for practising a therapy for which he had not received proper training but also for putting patients at risk by practising a totally unproven therapy, not supported by any evidence (Q 1053).

5.72 The GMC has guidelines on the position of medical practitioners wishing to refer patients to other practitioners and, although these guidelines are general, they expect doctors to observe them in relation to CAM referrals as with all other referrals: "Where doctors refer patients to an alternative or complementary practitioner, Good Medical Practice requires doctors to be satisfied that the healthcare workers concerned are accountable to a statutory regulatory body" (P 96). In terms of the position of a doctor who delegates treatment to a non-statutory regulated practitioner and still retains full responsibility for the patient's healthcare they explained: "...the doctor cannot delegate responsibility completely to another non-professional colleague but could delegate part of the treatment task to that individual. They retain overall responsibility for the care of the patient. I think, because of that, they have got to take great care in what they seek to delegate to someone else" (QQ 1059 & 1060).

5.73 The regulatory body for nurses, the United Kingdom Central Council for Nursing, Midwifery and Health Visiting (UKCC), told us that their members could practise CAM as long as they did so within the general guidelines on conduct and professional practice set out by the UKCC to apply to all nursing practice: "The UKCC believes that any registered practitioner who chooses to practise complementary therapies within their own sphere of practice should do so in accordance with the standards expected of that practitioner, and that is within the Code of professional conduct and by the principles laid out in the scope of professional practice. They indicate that if somebody is going beyond what their initial training encompassed, they should actually look at those principles to guide any further development" (Q 565). The UKCC do not issue specific guidelines on what training courses they consider are of an appropriate standard for nurses who want to learn about specific CAM therapies, but they did say that if a nurse practised a therapy for which they had "not sought the appropriate training" (Q 566) this could be considered a breach of the code of conduct.

5.74 The UKCC's emphasis is on nurses practising self-regulation and they offer very little specific guidance on which therapies are safe or appropriate or on where to train in specific therapies. Considering nurses are a group known often to practise CAM, especially those therapies in our Group 2, this seems to be an area where clear guidelines would be beneficial. However the UKCC did tell us: "We are responsive to the needs of people on our register and if we do receive a large number of enquiries from nurses etc. about this particular aspect...that is how we develop new guidance in response to their needs. So, yes, we would be prepared to consider guidance if the need was evident" (Q 585).

5.75 We also heard evidence about the regulation of veterinary surgeons wishing to practise CAM. The Royal College of Veterinary Surgeons pointed out that the Veterinary Surgeons Act 1966 limits the treatment of animals to qualified veterinary surgeons although others can treat animals under the direction of a veterinary surgeon who has examined the animal and prescribed the treatments (p 193). Thus they told us: "The underlying position is...that complementary and alternative treatments which amount to veterinary surgery are already subject to statutory regulation" (p 193). We also heard from the Association of British Veterinary Acupuncture which represents veterinarians who wish to practise acupuncture. They told us: "We believe that veterinary surgeons are the only people sufficiently qualified to really fully assess the health of any animal, to make a diagnosis about conditions, to formulate a treatment and to present a prognosis. This applies to conventional or complementary medicine. The principles of this are embodied in the Veterinary Surgeons Act, which gives us a rather nice monopoly to look after the welfare and health of animals in our care" (Q 807). Although the Association of British Veterinary Acupuncture is in a good position to advise veterinarians wishing to practise acupuncture, we heard no evidence that the Royal College of Veterinary Surgeons or any other veterinary body has issued formal guidelines for veterinarians wishing to practise CAM, or on relevant training courses, but informal guidelines are emerging.

5.76 The General Dental Council (GDC), the statutory body for the regulation of dentistry, told us that: "Dentists may be involved in complementary and alternative medicine in a number of ways. The Council would expect that at all times dentists would act in accordance with those sections of the Council's ethical guidance which have a bearing on these matters" (p 75). The ethical guidance to which this quotation refers is published in the Council's document *Maintaining Standards* which deals with issues such as acting in the patient's best interests, providing a high standard of care, the obligation to obtain patient consent and the seriousness of making misleading claims in relation to any treatment. However, it does not explicitly refer to complementary medicine at any time. The GDC told us: "The Council does not consider that this guidance needs amendment although it anticipates, in the light of greater public interest in complementary and alternative approaches, more discussion on these matters particularly in relation to the exercise of its jurisdiction" (p 76).

5.77 The evidence we have heard from the conventional medical, nursing, dental and veterinary regulatory bodies makes it clear that they all take quite a passive position on their members practising CAM. None of them has promulgated clear guidelines for their members who may be practising CAM. This means that the position of those working in these professions who wish to practise CAM is not very clear.

5.78 However, one body that has issued guidelines in this area is the BMA. In their document *New Approaches to Good Practice* they state: "Medically qualified practitioners wishing to practise any form of non-conventional therapy should take recognised training in the field approved by the appropriate regulatory body, and should only practise the therapies after registration"[41]. This is not at present practicable.

5.79 **We recommend that each existing regulatory body in the healthcare professions should develop clear guidelines on competency and training for their members on the position they take in relation to their members' activities in well organised CAM disciplines; as well as guidelines on appropriate training courses and other relevant issues. In drawing up such guidelines the conventional regulatory bodies should communicate with the relevant complementary regulatory bodies and the Foundation for Integrated Medicine to obtain advice on training and best practice and to encourage integrated practice.**

5.80 Although the main conventional regulatory bodies are not providing guidance for their members on CAM practice, there are some bodies which represent conventional practitioners who practise certain CAM therapies. The Faculty of Homeopathy is one such body representing medical practitioners who wish to incorporate homeopathy into their practice. The British Medical Acupuncture Society is a similar body representing medically qualified acupuncturists. These bodies provide an information resource for doctors interested in this area; they also run training courses specifically designed for medically qualified people wishing to train in the therapy in question. These bodies have a valuable role in promoting and regularising the position of CAM in the conventional medical world; however, it is not compulsory for conventional practitioners who practise CAM to be members of these bodies and they are not regulatory bodies (as their members are already regulated by the GMC or the UKCC).

5.81 One weakness in the current situation is the lack of communication between those bodies representing conventional medical practitioners who also practise specific CAM therapies and the CAM bodies representing individual therapies. This leads to little agreement on educational standards, little collaboration on research and, most worryingly, no clear agreement on information policies within a therapy to help the public understand their options when wishing to consult a practitioner of a particular therapy. For example, the British Medical Acupuncture Society told us that, although they are beginning to try and build bridges with the British Acupuncture Council (which represents non-medical acupuncturists), their meetings are at an "embryonic stage", and although they hope to discuss a way of helping the public understand their options this had not happened yet (Q 1021). In fact they told us that a member of the public might only distinguish between a medically qualified acupuncturist and a non-medical acupuncturist by "careful inquiry" and even then there may "still be some confusion" (QQ 1026 & 1027). Similarly the Faculty of Homeopathy told us there have not been any planned or significant discussions with the Society of Homoeopaths on giving the public clear advice on choosing a homeopath (Q 673).

---

[41] British Medical Association. *Complementary Medicine: New Approaches to Good Practice* (Oxford University Press, 1993).

5.82 We also heard from the bodies representing statutory regulated health professionals practising CAM about their attitude towards the level of training required of medically qualified personnel who wish to practise CAM therapies, in comparison to the level of training that should be required of non-medically qualified persons. The Faculty of Homeopathy told us that their core curriculum for training in the specialism of homeopathy has been developed independently of that of the Society of Homoeopaths because "we are not training the same people so a core curriculum for someone starting from scratch to become a homeopath is a completely different training pathway from the core curriculum for a doctor that has done undergraduate and postgraduate training" (Q 672). When we questioned them on which group was given more in-depth training on the principles of homeopathy itself (as opposed to physiology, research methods etc.) they said: "I think the membership exam in homeopathy in terms of homeopathic training for the homeopathic remedies, analysis and skill is probably similar to the Society of Homoeopaths" (Q 671).

5.83 **We would encourage the bodies representing medical and non-medical CAM therapists, particularly those in our Groups 1 and 2, to collaborate more closely, especially on developing reliable public information sources.** More collaboration on developing core curricula would be valuable, as it is important that both medically qualified and non-medically qualified practitioners are trained to the same level of skill in the therapy in question; sharing the knowledge of how to do this and spreading training resources will benefit both groups. **We recommend that if CAM is to be practised by any conventional healthcare practitioners, they should be trained to standards comparable to those set out for that particular therapy by the appropriate (single) CAM regulatory body**

5.84 The indemnification of medical practitioners and other health care professionals who wish to practise CAM is also an important issue. We were made aware of the guidance of the Medical Protection Society to its members on the use of CAM. This guidance is as follows:

"The Society recognises the benefits from bona fide complementary techniques and does not wish to inhibit members from providing treatments proven to be beneficial to patients.

"Practitioners should only undertake procedures which are in the patient's best interests and for which the practitioner has the requisite skill, training and facilities.

"In the event of any claim, complaint or other legal challenge the practitioner must be able to demonstrate that he or she was acting in accordance with recognised medical practice, and that experts in the field would support that form of management.

"The Society's Council considers it improper for practitioners to employ unproven or speculative techniques, and will not usually provide an indemnity in such circumstances. Council expects members of the Society to participate in continuing medical education to ensure that they remain fully up to date in their chosen areas of practice and participate in audit.

"Practitioners offering alternative forms of medicine should notify the Society of the technique employed within their practice and answer any supplementary questions. Withholding information or providing false or misleading answers, will usually disqualify the practitioner from any benefits of membership for incidents arising from any form of medical practice."

5.85 Under the Dentists Act, individuals are restricted as registered dentists to undertaking the business and practice of dentistry. Therefore in providing CAM as registered dentists this must only be done in conjunction with the practice of dentistry. Should a dentist offer CAM treatment outside the scope of the practice of dentistry, then he would not be providing it as a registered dentist and such treatment would not be covered by any indemnity offered by a protection organisation.

Regulation of Herbal Products

5.86 In evidence we have received, the regulation of herbal products has emerged as presenting particular challenges for public health. We have heard evidence that the use of herbal products makes up a significant proportion of the total consumption of medicines and other health products in the United Kingdom. The Pharmaceutical Society of Great Britain and the Proprietary Association of Great Britain told us that, while the total size of the market was difficult to estimate, in their view total annual sales of herbal products were between £93 million (for the retail sector) and up to £240 million per annum (including direct sales, Internet sales and mail order), with signs of continuing strong growth.

5.87 It was also evident that the regulation of these products is not satisfactory. The Department of Health told us that "...the present regulatory arrangements for herbal medicines have significant weaknesses. The regime for unlicensed herbal remedies does not provide sufficient protection or information for the public. At the same time, some of the regulatory hurdles for licensed medicines may be unnecessarily demanding for relatively benign herbal remedies" (P 108).

5.88 We heard evidence of the potential dangers that arise from inadequate regulation in this area. The Committee on Safety of Medicines (CSM), set up to provide advice to the Government's MCA, told us that in their opinion "the regulation of unlicensed herbal remedies is unsatisfactory and of considerable concern" (p 247). Evidence about the adulteration of various Chinese products with the toxic herb *Aristolochia* had led to sweeping restrictions on these products by MCA.

5.89 The formal position relating to herbal products was outlined for the European Union as a whole by the European Agency for the Evaluation of Medicinal Products (EMEA) based in London. The founding principles of medicines law, the basis formally of all ensuing legislation across all Member States of the European Union, are set out in European Council Directive 65/65/EEC. This defined medicinal products as "any substance or combination of substances, presented for treating or preventing disease in human beings or animals; or which may be administered with a view to making a medical diagnosis or to restoring, correcting or modifying physiological functions in human beings or animals." These definitions mean that any product that is supplied with therapeutic intent, for example by having a claim on the label, is a medicinal product and requires a licence (or marketing authorisation) in each Member State.

5.90 The EMEA has established a formal Working Party on Herbal Medicinal Products to advise it and the industry on harmonising licensing procedures for herbal medicinal products across the European Union. This has, among other activities, reviewed the application of European Union regulations on the licensing of herbal medicinal products, and considered the drafts of common standards for herbal medicinal products across the European Union, based on submissions to it of draft monographs by a scientific network: the European Scientific Cooperative on Phytotherapy (ESCOP) whose Chairman also gave evidence to us. It was clear to us from the latter that the supply of herbal products in much of the European Union is well integrated into conventional healthcare, with most herbs being supplied by pharmacists and many recommended or prescribed by physicians.

5.91 Especially in Germany, France, and the United Kingdom, a large number of herbal medicinal products have obtained marketing authorisations, under the terms of Directive 65/65/EEC. However most of these have been on the basis of historical licences of right awarded for products on the market when medicines legislation, such as the Medicines Act 1968 in the United Kingdom, came into force. We have heard that it has been extremely difficult for manufacturers of herbal products to achieve marketing authorisations for new products. As confirmed by the CSM, even a well-researched herb like St. John's Wort, with strong evidence for efficacy in depressive conditions, has not been licensed as a medicine in the United Kingdom. This means that the majority of herbal products, including almost all those originating from China, India and other non-European cultures, are not licensed as medicines and are supplied to the public without specific regulation. In the United Kingdom, the terms of the Medicines Act 1968 allow exemptions from licensing for a herbal remedy which is made up solely of the herb, and is supplied without recommendations as to its use. Thus St. John's Wort products are sold as remedies exempt from licensing, in spite of growing evidence of potential interactions with conventional medication. This exemption is not encountered elsewhere in the European Union, but this anomaly may well be corrected by forthcoming legislation.

5.92 It was generally apparent from evidence submitted, that as well as in the United Kingdom, there are significant inconsistencies in the application of medicines legislation to herbal products across the European Union. We heard further from the EMEA that these notably applied to defining the borderline between a medicine and a non-medicinal product such as a food or cosmetic: "...the choice and decision as to on which side of the borderline [a product lies] in principle is a decision for the Member State and the competent authority of that Member State. Understandably this leads to different decisions taken in different Member States. This is part of the confusion of herbal products today" (Q 125).

5.93 The difficulties faced by the public in identifying products that are adequately regulated were clearly demonstrated by the Proprietary Association of Great Britain (PAGB). They brought before us examples of similar proprietary health products available over the counter. Some were licensed as medicines by the MCA and thus met rigorous pharmaceutical standards of quality, safety and efficacy. Others, perhaps even produced by the same manufacturer, had no such licence and were not required to meet such standards. Only an inconspicuous licence number differentiated the two products. In the words of the PAGB, the consumer has "no way of knowing at all" (Q 1374) if a herbal or other natural product is licensed or unlicensed, sold as foods, or as exempt products. **We recommend that the MCA find a mechanism that would allow members of the public to identify health products that had met the stringent requirements of licensing and to differentiate them from unregulated competitors. This should be accompanied by strong enforcement of the law in regard to**

products that might additionally confuse the customer with claims and labelling that resemble those permitted by marketing authorisations.

5.94 Particular concern was raised about the import of herbal products from parts of the world where standards of quality might be harder to assure. The public in the United Kingdom consumes increasing quantities of herbal products from China, India and other parts of Asia, and Africa. The case of *Aristolochia* highlighted the difficulties in assuring quality where European Union regulations and audit procedures did not apply. We have also heard that herbal products from the USA are generally produced as dietary supplements without the regulatory controls applied to medicinal products.

5.95 In response to the increasing unease across the European Union about the inadequate regulation of herbal products, a working group was set up by the Pharmaceutical Committee of the European Commission. This Committee is currently considering draft proposals from the United Kingdom MCA for a new Directive for the regulation of herbal medicinal products, that would allow licensing of herbal medicines with evidence of traditional use, in lieu of new clinical or other evidence of efficacy, provided normal medicinal quality and safety standards are applied. We understand that the formal draft of such a Directive will be published around the time of our Report. **We strongly recommend that the Government should maintain their effective advocacy of such a new regulatory framework for herbal medicines in the United Kingdom and the rest of the European Union, and urge all parties to ensure that new regulations adequately reflect the complexities of the unregulated sector.**

5.96 We were encouraged that there was consensus that any new legislative framework for herbal medicinal products would remain within the framework of 65/65/EEC and subsequent medicines legislation, rather than in some less regulated environment. In particular all witnesses agreed that there could be no compromise with medicinal standards of quality for the regulation of herbal products. As the CSM put it, regulation should be "…based on the belief that good manufacturing practices are at the heart of the matter and that this is accepted by the industry and adopted. That the constituents, particularly, are authenticated carefully and that proof of product quality with appropriate specifications of both the raw materials and the finished products is available. There should be adequate testing to restrict the level of potentially hazardous constituents, and warnings about safe and correct use" (Q 1281).

5.97 Amongst our witnesses there was some debate, but no consensus, about the possibility of the United Kingdom developing national mechanisms for regulating the supply of herbal products if moves across the European Union were unsuccessful. The Proprietary Association of Great Britain considered that residual powers remained for effective regulation, without recourse to primary legislation. **We are concerned about the safety implications of an unregulated herbal sector and we urge that all legislative avenues be explored to ensure better control of this unregulated sector in the interests of the public health.**

5.98 We have also heard that many complementary practitioners use herbal products as part of their professional activities. The European Herbal Practitioners Association, which is co-ordinating a move among the professions towards statutory regulation for the herbal practitioner, told us that the major incentive for this move was to protect their role in law as suppliers of herbal medicinal products (Q 728). They also told us that they were concerned that too rigorous an application of medicines licensing requirement to their dispensing supplies could restrict their practice to untenable levels. **We support the view that any new regulatory regime should respect the diversity of products used by herbal practitioners and allow for simplified registration of practitioner stocks. Nevertheless, any such regime must ensure that levels of quality and assurance of safety are not compromised.**

CHAPTER 6: PROFESSIONAL TRAINING AND EDUCATION

Standards of CAM Training Courses

6.1 High quality, accredited training of practitioners in the principal CAM disciplines is vital in ensuring that the public are protected from incompetent and dangerous practitioners. Evidence we have received has indicated that CAM training courses vary in their content, depth and duration, both between disciplines and in some cases within the same discipline. FIM articulated this in their written evidence: "There is great variation in the standards of the many CAM training institutions. Training for some therapies i.e. acupuncture, chiropractic, herbal medicine, homeopathy and osteopathy is highly developed with degree level courses that are externally validated. For others, arrangements are not as advanced" (P 88). Of course, with the wide range of disciplines that exist within CAM, not all therapies require or are equally capable of supporting intensive training, but even within the same therapeutic disciplines training standards vary from course to course.

6.2 There seems to be a consensus across CAM and conventional medical bodies that responsibility for training standards and the validation of training should lie with the appropriate CAM professional regulatory body. Evidence also indicates that therapies furthest down the path towards achieving a single professional regulatory body are those with the most developed educational structures.

6.3 The study on the CAM professional organisations, referred to in paragraph 1.16, examined each organisation's training standards[42]. This was carried out first in 1997 and repeated in 2000. The study was based on a questionnaire designed to elicit the "current status, activities and aspirations" of professional associations in the CAM fields and included questions on the entry and educational requirements for each CAM professional body. With regard to educational standards four questions were asked:

(i) whether a formal accreditation procedure was used to screen the membership;

(ii) whether the members were required to graduate from an accredited and/or recognised college;

(iii) whether members were required to participate in Continuing Professional Development;

(iv) what minimum length of study was required to be eligible for membership.

6.4 The following pages refer to the data extracted from the responses to these questions. Mills and Budd, the authors, note that in the absence of formal regulatory structures for CAM very little of the information is independently accredited. They also advocate caution about interpreting these data. In response to the first question, if an organisation claims to have a formal accreditation procedure to guide entry it may imply little more than the existence of certain procedural requirements that their members must fulfil. Organisations that do not have such mechanisms may have a 'default' route for members who have graduated from a specific institution to which the organisation is linked. If this is the case the organisation should answer positively to question two. If they do not respond positively to question (i) or (ii) this may mean they do not operate rigorous membership requirements.

6.5 Mills and Budd also note that if an organisation answers positively in response to question two, this may mean they have a close link to the training establishment out of which they were founded, and may not yet have managed to become independent of that establishment. This is common in some CAM disciplines because training courses were often established before a professional body existed; graduates from particular colleges often then started a professional body and operated it as a facility for students from that institution.

6.6 The provision of Continuing Professional Development could be regarded as a sign of a discipline's maturity. A positive answer to the third question, however, would not necessarily indicate how much Continuing Professional Development the organisation advocates, or whether it is a mandatory requirement for membership: the Exeter authors' experience indicates the latter is rare.

6.7 Finally Mills and Budd express concern over interpreting data given on "minimum hours required for training"; the answers provided are not the result of an accreditation process and, thus, can only provide a sketchy idea of the range of requirements across organisations; hence such figures as are available are unreliable.

6.8 Using the Exeter Report and the evidence made available to us by several witnesses we have attempted to illustrate the variations in training provision in the CAM sector.

---

[42] Mills, S. & Budd, S. (2000) (*Op. cit.*).

TRAINING IN STATUTORILY REGULATED CAM THERAPIES

6.9 Osteopathy and chiropractic, the two CAMs with professional bodies established by statute, have clear guidelines on education set by their respective regulatory councils (the General Osteopathic Council, GOsC, and the General Chiropractic Council, GCC). The GOsC and the GCC also have the advantage that by law all those practitioners calling themselves osteopaths or chiropractors must abide by the training standards set by the respective regulatory bodies. Practitioners of mainstream osteopathy, chiropractic, acupuncture, medical homeopathy and herbal medicine now recognise their limits of competence and will refer patients whose problems do not lie within those limits, for conventional medical treatment. It is worth reflecting on how the GOsC and the GCC have implemented the validation of their training standards.

6.10 The GOsC explained that they have been working on improving and validating the training courses for future osteopathic students and on validating the training and competence of existing osteopaths who wish to continue to practise and so have to register with the new GOsC (Q 456). They explained that they had embarked on a "recognised qualification process as laid down in the Osteopaths Act". This involved asking each training provider to "map their provision, their profile and their resources, and in particular their clinical education provision". Of the thirteen educational providers that existed at the beginning of the process, seven have been deemed satisfactory.

6.11 The GOsC also explained that the Osteopaths Act allows them to raise the standard of proficiency required to graduate as an osteopath. Their current standard of proficiency, which provides minimum standards of competence through which to assess students, was developed by the King's Fund Working Party on Osteopathy, chaired by Sir Thomas (now Lord) Bingham. They have now consulted with the osteopathic training providers and these standards are currently in the process of being upgraded. They are developing a number of quality assurance mechanisms to ensure that training remains at a high standard and will use external examiners to monitor the final assessment of students; they are also continually monitoring standards.

6.12 In assessing the training and competence of existing osteopaths who wished to register with the GOsC, they concluded that "…it was not appropriate to rely on the retrospective recognition of qualifications in osteopathy as a means test of entry to the statutory register for practising osteopaths" (p 99). This was partly due to training in the area having previously been delivered in a wide variety of ways with no common curriculum, and partly because many institutions that had provided osteopathic qualifications now no longer exist (Q 444). As a consequence of this the GOsC have developed a comprehensive standard of proficiency and a strict registering system whereby all existing osteopaths have to provide evidence that they were sufficiently trained by submitting to scrutiny a "Professional Profile and Portfolio".

6.13 The professional profile and portfolio asks each individual to "…provide evidence to support his or her claim to have practised to an adequate level of safety and osteopathic competence within the prescribed timeframe of the Act" (Q 444). Ms Sarah Wallace, Acting Chairman of the GOsC education committee, believes that the professional profile and portfolio offers individual applicants from diverse backgrounds "the means to make realistic and verifiable claims" that they meet the standard of proficiency. She also explained that the portfolio required each individual to reflect in detail on their training and practice as well as on their future training, practice and intentions for engaging in Continuing Professional Development.

6.14 The GCC have approached the validation process in a slightly different way (and because of the later enactment of the Chiropractors Act their progress is slightly behind that of the GOsC). Like the GOsC, the GCC have Standards of Safe and Competent Practice for Chiropractors as well as published Standards of Education (Q 478). They have an accreditation process for chiropractic training providers consistent with that of other professional groups, in that it requires certain documents to be presented and site-visits to each institution to talk to staff and students (Q 493). In terms of validating the training of existing practitioners, the GCC differ from the GOsC in relying on the retrospective recognition of qualifications. To this end they ask each applicant for a detailed Curriculum Vitae. They also check the applicant's insurance history, and search for any evidence of a criminal record, etc. (Q 477).

6.15 However the GCC are currently working on developing their educational structure in two other important areas. Firstly they are looking into establishing a pre-registration year of practice after training, before students become fully registered (Q 485). Secondly they are consulting the profession and the public on what form a scheme of Continuing Professional Development should take. Their Act allows them to specify that a certain amount of Continuing Professional Development should be undertaken and they will be exercising that power in due course (Q 505).

6.16 The GCC is less advanced along the path of developing educational standards than the GOsC are, and the two bodies have taken different routes towards educational validation. It is too early in the respective lives of these Councils to judge the relative success of their approaches to educational validation. However, both bodies have interesting elements in their requirements which look promising. We are interested in the GCC's moves towards establishing a supervised pre-registration year of practice, similar to the pre-registration year of medical training under supervision, which may be considered as a model for other therapies, specifically those in our Group 1.

TRAINING IN NON-STATUTORILY REGULATED CAM THERAPIES

6.17 Training standards in the non-statutory regulated CAMs vary widely, usually in proportion to the level of professional development within the particular CAM discipline. Those therapies which are closest to achieving a single regulatory body to represent all therapists in the field are most likely to have clearly defined training standards. A number of therapies' training standards are reviewed below, by way of example, to illustrate the variations that exist. Those disciplines which are not reviewed here have very variable, often limited, training programmes.

Current Status of Training

6.18 *Acupuncture* – We received evidence from the British Acupuncture Council. The Exeter Report[43] describes the British Acupuncture Council as the largest group representing acupuncturists in the United Kingdom and as having 'led the way among complementary professions in establishing verifiable standards of education for their profession.' The British Acupuncture Council has been involved in the formation of an Independent Accreditation Board for Educational Standards. This was established to ensure that no college or course would be advocated by the Council without being scrutinised by an independent board, which has an independent Chair and 16 members from a range of professions (pp 28 & 29). The Council explained why establishing the Accreditation Board was such an important step: "When the British Acupuncture Accreditation Board was first created the profession was quite fragmented. There were five professional associations. Although they met in the Council for Acupuncture and were able to agree some things together, like a common code of ethics and a code of practice, they were not able to agree a core curriculum for educational standards. This was partly because, at the time, schools which were working as commercial private enterprises emphasised their differences more than the common features they shared. Therefore, that was one of the most difficult things for us to establish: a dialogue and agreement over educational standards. We felt that creating an independent board was the best way to overcome these difficulties. The board has been immensely useful in helping facilitate the process of peer review, which the profession at the time was fairly nervous about. Also, it helped to develop a consensus producing a common core curriculum" (Q 765).

6.19 The British Acupuncture Council are already looking at ways to move forward by "...looking at a change in the relationship between the Board and the British Acupuncture Council, partly as a result of discussions with the Department of Health, who are recommending that accreditation should be managed by an accreditation committee which reports directly to the governing body. The British Acupuncture Council must be fully accountable for all its educational processes. This is in line with what has been established for the osteopaths and chiropractors. So we are now looking at setting up this kind of structure. We believe the processes and procedures of accreditation have been exemplary and we would not like to change these" (Q765).

6.20 The problems highlighted by the British Acupuncture Council, which show why it was important for them to set up an independent accreditation board, are ones we have found to be common across the CAM professions. Fragmentation, disagreement between groups and concentration on differences rather than common aims are frequent problems. **Establishing an independent accreditation board along the lines of the British Acupuncture Accreditation Board is a positive move. Other therapies with fragmented professional representation may wish to use this as a model.**

6.21 *Homeopathy* – In Mills & Budd's survey four organisations representing non-medically qualified homeopaths were identified. Only one of these used a formal accreditation process to screen membership, although all required members to graduate from a professional college and all required continuing professional education. The Exeter study found that the minimum educational criteria used by these organisations ranged from three years of full-time to three years of part-time study. The largest homeopathic professional organisation, the Society of Homoeopaths, told us about their work with "the other smaller bodies which also represent homeopaths in this country" to develop National

---

[43]   Mills, S. & Budd, S. (2000) *(Op. cit.).*

Occupational Standards in homeopathy with the assistance of Healthwork UK (see paras 5.56 – 5.63). The Society of Homoeopaths explained how they have used these to enhance their education policy: "We almost immediately began to use the National Occupational Standards in several areas. Throughout our educational policy document we refer to the National Occupational Standards when we are examining the criteria presented by the course providers who meet our recognised criteria for our educational policy" (Q 681). The merits of National Occupational Standards are discussed in paragraphs 6.63 – 6.70.

6.22 The development of National Occupational Standards has benefited the Society. The joint work involved in developing the standards has had other benefits in developing the professional structure of homeopathy. The Society and the other smaller bodies "...have recently got together to form a common council and our objective is to move forward using these competencies to establish a national register for homeopathic practitioners with all the requisite infrastructure for that. When we have achieved that stage of development we will then carefully consider the next possible option which will be that of statutory self-regulation" (Q 676).

6.23 The Society told us that they felt their educational requirements were progressing well. "There has been quite a development in education...things have evolved in the last 22 years quite dramatically; during that time we have seen the introduction of full-time courses equivalent to undergraduate degree training. We now have two university degrees, BSc (Hons) degrees in homeopathic education. The interesting thing about these degrees is that the conventional medical part of the education, which contains basic anatomy, physiology, pathology, research methodology etc., is part of the curriculum which has been written by doctors" (Q 677).

6.24 *Herbalism* – We heard evidence from the European Herbal Practitioners Association (EHPA) which was established in 1993 to unify the herbal medicine profession. It has been working towards bringing herbal practitioners from a variety of different backgrounds under one body with a common core curriculum (P 78). They explained that their core curriculum lays down basic standards of training and is 'science based', in that it teaches the basics of conventional medicine and points out the limits of competence of trained herbalists. To reflect the growing number of BSc degree programmes available in this subject, the core curriculum is aimed at a four-year university course. However at the time of their giving evidence, the core curriculum was not yet in force although they had just launched an independent accreditation board to make sure educational providers measure up to this standard (QQ 705-711). Mills and Budd's study found that the educational requirements for membership in the herbal medicine organisations ranged from 4 years of full-time study to 2 years of part-time study. The EHPA's desire to undergo statutory regulation may provide a future body which can reconcile such differences.

6.25 *Nutritional Therapy* – The Nutritional Therapy Council (established in 1999) is an umbrella body for the nutritional therapists, which focuses particularly on educational standards and on developing National Occupational Standards for the profession. The largest nutritional therapy organisation is the British Association of Nutritional Therapists. They believe that the Nutritional Therapy Council will be able to co-ordinate training colleges. Currently educational requirements for membership of the different nutritional therapy bodies range from 4 years full-time to 2 years part-time. All bodies require members to graduate from a recognised college, and over half use the formal accreditation process to screen membership. However, fewer than half require Continuing Professional Development for their members.

6.26 *Aromatherapy* – We heard from the Aromatherapy Organisations Council who told us that they represent the 'majority of professionally qualified aromatherapists' who work in the field of complementary medicine, through their 12 professional member associations. The therapists recognised by the Council have trained to standards defined in that body's core curriculum (P 9). Mills & Budd identified 12 organisations that represented aromatherapists, but all came under the umbrella body of the Aromatherapy Organisations Council, and were working towards the same core curriculum. The Aromatherapy Organisations Council's minimum educational requirement for membership is nine months part-time which adds up to 180 hours, plus 50 supervised treatment hours.

6.27 *Massage* – Mills & Budd's study emphasised that there are many types of massage, some of which fall within the spectrum of beauty therapy; those they surveyed emphasised the health effects of massage. The study identified nine organisations representing massage therapists but noted that many massage therapists may also be members of aromatherapy organisations as the two therapies are often practised together. The proportion of massage therapists in organisations that use a formal accreditation process to screen membership was found to be small but all required members to graduate from a recognised college and almost all required continuing professional education. For membership the time committed to educational requirements ranged from 1600 hours to 100 hours.

6.28 *Reflexology* – Mills & Budd's study identified ten bodies representing reflexologists. Most practitioners were in organisations that used a formal accreditation process to screen membership, all requiring members to graduate from a recognised college; but fewer than half such organisations required Continuing Professional Development. Educational requirements for membership ranged from 60 to 100 hours of training. Recently all the reflexology organisations identified have agreed to work together within a new reflexology forum, launched in September 2000, towards identifying new National Occupational Standards for the discipline.

6.29 *Shiatsu* – Mills & Budd's study identified five organisations representing Shiatsu practitioners in the United Kingdom. This was considered to be a retrogressive step as in 1997 nearly all practitioners had been represented by one body. However, all the organisations identified used a formal accreditation process and required members to graduate from a recognised college. They also found that most required some form of Continuing Professional Development. The educational requirements for membership varied between 150 to 500 hours of training.

6.30 *Healing* – Mills & Budd's study identified twelve organisations representing registered healers; most, but not all, of these have accepted the authority of the Confederation of Healing Organisations. The educational requirement for that Confederation is either 2 years' full-time training or one year part-time. However it does not use a formal accreditation process to screen for membership, it does not require members to have graduated from a recognised college nor does it require continuing professional education. For those practitioners in groups outside the Confederation most use a formal accreditation process to screen membership and most require Continuing Professional Development. The educational requirements of these other bodies vary enormously from 2 days' to 2 years' part-time training.

6.31 *Alexander Technique* – Mills & Budd's study identified three Alexander Technique associations. However, unlike other groups within the complementary and alternative sector, the Alexander Technique professionals consider themselves as teachers rather than healthcare practitioners. Each of these groups uses a formal accreditation process to screen membership but does not require members to have graduated from a recognised college. Continuing Professional Development is usually required. The educational requirement for membership ranges from 3 years' full-time to 4 years' part-time training.

General Conclusions

6.32 FIM has used Mills and Budd's report to draw conclusions about the status of CAM education in the United Kingdom: "The report by the University of Exeter suggests that the CAM professions should engage in vigorous attempts to reassure the public that their training courses are sound, validated and consistent and that they incorporate modern experience of health and illness, as well as more established teaching techniques. It is important in this context that CAM practitioners, teachers and researchers also understand the advantages of more systematic audit and rigorous research within their practice" (P 88). Currently it is legal for anyone in the United Kingdom to practise any CAM therapy without having ever had any relevant training, except in the cases of osteopathy and chiropractic (which are protected by statute). This is disquieting; fortunately this does not seem to be a common problem but it does remain a possibility for all the therapies that are not so protected.

6.33 **We recommend that CAM training courses should become more standardised and be accredited and validated by the appropriate professional bodies. All those who deliver CAM treatments, whether conventional health professionals or CAM professionals, should have received training in that discipline independently accredited by the appropriate regulatory body.** This was the view expressed by the Department of Health, and we agree (P 111). This would protect the public who use CAM and would improve the transparency of the organisations and make understanding what practitioners' qualifications mean easier. It is clear to us that the quality and degree of standardisation of training within each therapy are closely linked to how successful each individual therapy has been in overcoming internal divisions and coming together under the auspices of a single body that agrees core objectives for education and regulation. The efforts of organisations such as the British Acupuncture Council to form an independent accreditation board must be commended and could be used as an example in related CAM fields. Improving training through the appropriate self-regulating body is an expressed aim of the Department of Health: "The Government's overall concern is to ensure that all those who deliver CAM treatments, whether orthodox health professionals or CAM professionals, should have received training in that discipline independently accredited by the appropriate CAM self-regulatory body" (P 111). We agree.

CONTINUING PROFESSIONAL DEVELOPMENT

6.34 Continuing Professional Development is uncommon in all CAMs. The public interest demands a better structure in the principal CAM disciplines. Even those from whom we have received evidence in the professions we included in Group 1 have uneven Continuing Professional Development requirements. Continuing Professional Development is vital if professionals are to keep up with new developments in their field; it is also a mechanism that can be used to encourage research understanding and inter-professional collaboration. We recognise that developing a coherent Continuing Professional Development structure to cover a whole profession requires the body in charge of such a scheme to devote considerable time and resources which some of the smaller CAM therapy professional bodies may find hard. However, there does seem to be a lack of keenness in some therapies to try to overcome such problems. **We suggest that the CAM therapies, particularly those in our Groups 1 and 2, should identify Continuing Professional Development in practice as a core requirement for their members.**

VALIDATION OF TRAINING

6.35 The accreditation and validation of training courses by the appropriate professional body is vital in ensuring their adequacy. It is important to note that a distinction exists between academic qualifications on the one hand and the ability either to practise or to register as a practitioner on the other.

6.36 The increasing availability of CAM training within higher educational institutions is an encouraging development, as it provides externally validated educational achievements. However there is some concern that even courses within universities, designed to train students to practise, are often not accredited by a professional regulatory body of the therapy being studied.

6.37 The Committee of Vice Chancellors and Principals (CVCP) explained, in relation to undergraduate qualifying courses, the difference between academic qualifications in a discipline and a license to practise that discipline: "In any area where a qualification is giving a licence to practise, whether in health or outside health, the university does not have the authority to award the licence to practise…Therefore, in those professions where there is an existing regulatory body such as the GMC, the Council for Professions Supplementary to Medicine or the UKCC…the universities do work very closely with the regulatory body that has the authority in the end to confer the licence to practise. The quality assurance regimes which underpin the programmes are commonly now run as an integrated set of activities with the universities' own quality assurance, with the academic stream or the academic qualification being integrated, in so far as it is possible, with the regulatory body's inspections of its interests…It follows from that situation that [even] where there is no regulatory body with the authority to give a license to practise the university cannot award the licence to practise" (Q 275). This statement does not, however, take into account the common position where universities have to work with the non-statutory regulated registering bodies which generally represent CAM therapies.

6.38 Many of the main CAMs now taught at university level have reasonably well-developed voluntary self-regulatory bodies with which the universities should liaise when setting standards. This is already happening in some cases. For example, the University of Westminster Centre for Community Care and Primary Health offers BSc degrees in several of the most popular CAM therapies. One of their objectives is "to collaborate with training organisations and professional bodies in developing educational programmes." This is a principle that we believe all CAM training courses should accept (P 235).

6.39 The Department of Health also share this view. They told us that "…in the most established of the CAM professions the regulatory body is responsible for the accreditation of training for the purposes of a licence to practise. Through its support for initiatives in relation to integrated medicine, the Department is encouraging developments in the accreditation of training systems throughout the whole of the CAM field" (Q 2).

6.40 **We consider that it is imperative that higher educational institutions and any regulatory bodies in CAM liaise in order to ensure that training is adequate for registration. If extra training is required after academic qualification to ensure fitness to practise, this should be defined by the appropriate professional body, which should then implement appropriate mechanisms in order to see that this objective is achieved.** One good example of this principle is that of the chiropractors who propose a pre-registration year of clinical practice which will be supervised. This is a principle which the main CAM therapies may wish to consider.

WHAT SHOULD CAM TRAINING COURSES INCLUDE?

Basics of Biomedical Science

6.41 It was a recommendation of several witnesses including FIM, the University of Westminster and the BMA, that CAM practitioners should be taught basic principles of anatomy and physiology as provided in orthodox healthcare training. The BMA stated that "all practices claiming therapeutic benefits should include in their training courses a foundation in the basic medical sciences" (P 45).

6.42 Most CAMs within our Group 1, which have established core curricula, include in their courses such basic knowledge as requirements set by their professional bodies.

6.43 **We recommend that training in anatomy, physiology and basic biochemistry and pharmacology should be included within the education of practitioners of therapies that are likely to offer diagnostic information, such as the therapies in Groups 1 and 3a. Although it may be useful for other therapists to understand basic biomedical science, there is no requirement for such in-depth understanding if the therapy being practised is to be used as an adjunct to conventional medicine.** This requirement should be tailored depending upon the limits of competence of each discipline

Research Methods

6.44 A theme that has repeated itself throughout this Inquiry is the lack of research into complementary medicine. The Research Council for Complementary Medicine (RCCM) referred to some evidence to support this perception: "Smaller studies carried out by a large number of independent clinics and units do not hide the fact that as yet there is only a limited research ethic among CAM practitioners in the UK" (P 180). Common reasons we were given for this were lack of understanding of research ethics and methodology among many CAM practitioners, a lack of willingness to evaluate evidence in order to change practice and a shortage of resources.

6.45 One reason for the poor research ethic among many CAM therapists is that many have never been trained in research methods or the importance of evidence-based practice. As a result, many CAM therapists are unable to take the opportunities of practice-based research and even fewer consider the opportunity of becoming an active researcher. Most medical and health-related research is undertaken by conventional healthcare practitioners or scientists with priorities that primarily emanate from the conventional medical domain. It is our opinion that until CAM undergraduates and practitioners become familiar with what research can offer and with the methods used to investigate processes and health outcomes, difficulties will continue to arise between those who will only accept CAM practice if it conforms to the rigours of conventional research requirements, and those in the CAM world who regard such scrutiny as irrelevant.

6.46 This is a view supported by many witnesses from whom we have heard. For example, in their written evidence to us the BMA state that: "Active support is needed for therapists embarking on research projects, including appropriate training in research techniques...Core curricula for undergraduate training establishments should include components on research methodology, information technology, and statistics" (P 44). They suggest "...training in clinical audit should also be provided, so that the practice and management of patients are evaluated rigorously at regular intervals" (P 45). Many submissions, including that from the University of Westminster (P 236), have highlighted the need for this problem to be addressed through incorporating research methods and statistics modules into CAM undergraduate courses. The CVCP indicated that they would expect any CAM courses taught in universities to include research methods: "Any university course worth the name nowadays has to have an evidence-based, self-critical, reflective element within it" (Q 280). Therefore they would "take it as given" that university courses should include proper research training within their curricula.

6.47 The RCCM supported the view that such education would help improve the overall picture of CAM research. They stated that "...a programme of research awareness for practitioners of complementary and alternative medicine would help improve the quality of research" (P 180).

6.48 If research training is incorporated into the curriculum of all CAM training courses, as we hope it will be, this should eventually lead to a new cadre of research-aware CAM practitioners, but such a development will take time. For a more immediate solution it would seem wise for existing practitioners to gain some research training. This would require initiatives to help practitioners cover the costs, and incentives to make them aware of the need. We asked the Department of Health if they had any initiative relating to making available training in research methods for practitioners who are keen to improve the evidence base of their profession; one of the Department of Health officials responded in the affirmative: "To give an example, until May of last year I was Regional Director of

Research and Development (R&D) for Trent region. We had within our regional R&D budget a substantial proportion of funding going into the provision of training for research work, most of it directly through the Trent Institute. That provided courses for practitioners in any field who wished to acquire skills, for example in statistics, epidemiology, research design and so on, which are the common tools, as it were, of research" (Q 18). This is quite a limited initiative but is a good example of how, at a regional level, it is possible to encourage practitioners to become interested in research. It is important that such initiatives are made more widely available and are publicised well. Informing the appropriate professional bodies of such initiatives and encouraging them to pass on the information to their practitioners would be a step in the right direction.

6.49 We recommend that that every therapist working in CAM should have a clear understanding of the principles of evidence-based medicine and healthcare. This should be a part of the curriculum of all CAM therapy courses. An in-depth understanding of research methods may be even more important for those therapies that operate independently of medical supervision, and which attempt to make a diagnosis and to cure complaints rather than for those which offer relaxation or aim to improve the general quality of life of patients. Therefore training in research and statistical methods may be particularly appropriate for practitioners of therapies in Groups 1 and 3a. But we consider that an understanding of research methods and outcomes should be included in the training of all CAM practitioners. It is important that all of those teaching these courses should understand these principles. Chapter 7 considers research training for CAM professionals in more detail.

Limits of Competence

6.50 A number of witnesses have emphasised the importance of CAM practitioners being aware of the limits of their competence and of when it is in the best interests of the patient to refer to other health-care professionals who are better qualified to deal with specific problems. The BMA stated that this should be an element of training: "Limits of competence must be established for each therapy during the training process. Patients suffering from conditions not amenable to treatment must be identified and referred to the appropriate agency. This is particularly important in cases where medical attention is needed" (P 45).

6.51 Many therapies do already consider the limits of their practitioners' competence in their training and in their code of ethics. For example the Society of Homoeopaths told us that bounds of competence "...is an issue we have taken to heart and have addressed in our code of ethics and practice. It is also an issue we have addressed with our member practitioners and an issue that has been taken into homeopathic colleges" (Q 868).

6.52 It is possible to argue that until more research on the efficacy of each therapy is done, it is hard to define the limits of competence of that therapy. **We recommend that all CAM training defines limits of the particular therapist's competence as clearly as possible in the state of current knowledge. Training should also give students clear guidance on when a patient should be referred to a primary care physician or even directly to secondary hospital care.**

Familiarisation With Other CAM Therapies

6.53 Evidence from many CAM associations has highlighted the importance of CAM practitioners being given CAM familiarisation courses so that they are aware of the other forms of treatment their patients may be accessing. However, few of our witnesses have suggested that such familiarisation should cover the whole spectrum of CAM. It is quite likely that patients accessing one type of CAM may also be accessing another and, as we have discussed previously, there is such a wide range of CAM professions that it is not necessarily true that a practitioner trained in one CAM discipline will know about all the others. An example emerged in the GCC's evidence when they explained that "...the position of complementary and alternative therapies has not been built into our training... other than as how to conduct oneself as a professional with other people who may be co-operating in the treatment: therapies like aromatherapy or crystal therapy and meditation are not things that crop up to any degree. I think there is a limit to what one can do within chiropractic education" (QQ 490 & 491).

6.54 We recommend that all CAM therapists should be made aware of the other CAM therapies available to their patients and how they are practised. We do not think it should be assumed that CAM practitioners competent in one discipline necessarily understand the others. When we visited the Southampton University Medical School we noted that the CAM familiarisation course available to medical undergraduates was also open to nurses and to students from the Anglo-European College of Chiropractic in Bournemouth. This enabled students to become familiar with CAM while meeting practitioners involved in different fields, sharing resources and encouraging interdisciplinary understanding and co-operation.

A Core Curriculum?

6.55 Some of our witnesses consider that a common core curriculum for all CAM training courses is needed to ensure that all therapies have a common awareness of the issues central to all forms of practice in healthcare. The BMA, FIM and the University of Westminster propose a core that embraces some or all of the following themes:

- Basic biomedicine;

- Fundamentals of conventional medical diagnosis and guidelines of patient referral;

- CAM therapies and their potential uses, including the principles of diagnosis and practice;

- Research methodology and the application of results;

- Holistic models of healthcare;

- Professional ethics;

- The therapeutic relationship;

- Clinical audit of outcomes;

- Impact of social, cultural, economic, employment and environmental factors on health;

- Counselling skills;

- Principles of quality management and audit;

- Organisational skills including record keeping;

- Technical skills including IT management etc.

6.56 This requirement may well depend on increasing partnerships being developed between medical schools and the newer universities.

6.57 If each of the principal complementary therapies develops one professional regulatory body responsible for supervising all training in that discipline, as we hope they will, this should result in core competencies being defined. These competencies will vary according to the extent to which the therapy claims to make independent diagnoses or is independent of medical supervision. Nevertheless, an understanding of the ethical aspects of healthcare, clinical audit and the therapeutic relationship should be part of all such training.

6.58 The University of Westminster, which offers several CAM courses, suggests that the advantages of a core curriculum are that it establishes the generic field of knowledge and skills required by such CAM practitioners, while also promoting inter-disciplinary learning and multi-disciplinary practice (P 236).

6.59 Although many witnesses have supported a core curriculum with similar components, there is less consensus over the professions to which it should extend. FIM's outline for a core curriculum is one which they see extending to the training of all healthcare professionals in all institutions (P 88). They promote a core curriculum applicable to all types of CAM, as well as to conventional practice because they see there being "a core body of knowledge that both CAM and orthodox practitioners need to understand" (Q 101). Their proposals are supported by others including the British Complementary Medicine Association (P 34).

6.60 However, several witnesses have objected to the idea of core curricula and their objections have mostly followed one of two arguments: either they believe that the range of CAM disciplines is so diverse that to envisage a common body of knowledge useful for them all is too difficult, or they disagree, *a priori,* on theoretical grounds with the concept of core curricula. The second objection was typified by the CVCP who told us: "It would not be the Committee of Vice Chancellors and Principals' position to advocate that a national core curriculum should be prescribed in any particular field of any sort. That is not something that the Committee of Vice Chancellors and Principals would embrace" (Q 277). They went on to suggest that it is the role of each therapy's regulatory body to prescribe outcomes of training: "In these particular areas both of western medicine and CAM it is clearly the case that the activity of the professional and regulatory bodies does prescribe something which may look more or less like a core curriculum, depending on the discipline". But although the CVCP support the idea of the regulatory bodies prescribing outcomes in this way they also support the need to "...give some flexibility to the individual universities to decide how to educate that practitioner so as to arrive at those desired outcomes".

6.61 **We conclude that there should be flexibility for training institutions to decide how to educate practitioners.** To introduce one formal core curriculum across healthcare would be a

Herculean task; there is no obvious body available to tackle such a task which, in any case, would no doubt meet with much opposition. We endorse the view of the CVCP (shared by many other witnesses) that **it is the relevant professional regulatory body of a specific CAM therapy that should set objectives of training and define core competencies appropriate to their particular discipline, and we so recommend. We do not advocate a blanket core curriculum.**

6.62 However, we do recommend that, whether subject to statutory or voluntary regulation, all healthcare regulatory bodies should consider the relevance to their respective professions of those elements set out above in paragraph 6.55.

NATIONAL OCCUPATIONAL STANDARDS

6.63 Setting training standards is an important step in protecting the public from inadequately trained practitioners and, as we have discussed, setting such standards is a role for each appropriate professional body. The Department of Health stated that the Government's position is that a pre-condition of membership of any professional register should be to meet recognised and appropriate standards of training set by the respective registering body. This is an integral part of professional regulation (P 110). However, considering that many of the CAM professions are fragmented, an outside body could work with the various CAM bodies to develop appropriate core training standards that would apply across each discipline.

6.64 In 1998, the Government approved the establishment of Healthwork UK, a new National Training Organisation set up to work with the Government and the healthcare sector in the field of education and training. The Department of Health see Healthwork UK's role as being to promote the development of individuals and to "assist in delivering Government training and development policies" (P 110). They state that one of the specific functions of Healthwork UK is to "support the needs of CAM practitioners by helping members of professions to work together to set standards of practice, education and training" (P 100).

6.65 We have heard evidence about the experience of working with Healthwork UK in developing National Occupational Standards from the homeopaths, one of the CAM groups to have recently developed National Occupational Standards. The National Occupational Standards for homeopathy were developed in collaboration by the Society of Homoeopaths, the Faculty of Homeopathy and several other homeopathic bodies. Both the Society and the Faculty told us that they felt the National Occupational Standards were a major leap forward (QQ 676 and 663). Undertaking this exercise with an independent organisation like Healthwork UK has helped to bring the various fragmented and disparate homeopathic associations together. Mr Stephen Gordon, Director of Political and NHS Affairs at the Society of Homoeopaths, said: "For us this marks a watershed and I am pleased to say that through the joint work involved in developing the National Occupational Standards, the Society, together with the other smaller bodies which also represent homeopaths in this country, has recently got together to form a common Council and our objective is to move forward these competencies to establish a single national register for homeopathic practitioners with all the requisite infrastructure for that" (Q 676). The Society also explained that they see the National Occupational Standards as having a key role in all three levels of training, registration and practice (Q 681).

6.66 The Faculty of Homeopathy, representing statutory registered doctors, point out that its members are not subject to the training requirements prescribed by the National Occupational Standards but they were still involved in their preparation. The Faculty echoed the Society's sentiments by saying that National Occupational Standards have "enabled the emerging profession of the homeopathic practitioner, which is currently unregulated, to define much more clearly what their job is and what their skills are. I think this will lead to a single register and maybe then consequently to statutory regulations" (Q 665).

6.67 We also asked Healthwork what benefits they saw for CAM therapies in developing National Occupational Standards under their guidance. They echoed the homeopaths' belief that they can help professions come together and defined this as a key role they play: "One of our roles is that we bring stakeholders together, we bring the educationalists together, the practitioners, we bring people offering courses together with those that need them, we bring members of the public into the debate. It really is useful to be able to say that at the end of all this effort you can say you have kite mark qualifications, you have kite mark standards behind them, the public safety is something demonstrable, the value for money associated with Government public funds going into this is demonstrable. The workforce which develops is evidentially a workforce which is developing with a view to patients getting better outcomes" (Q 1456).

6.68 Healthwork also told us that they felt they could be of particular benefit to CAM bodies not only as an outside unifying force but also because they themselves have a good system of support both in terms of regulation and finance, which much of CAM lacks: "We are supported by the Education Act regulatory authorities. We have access to funds as a National Training Organisation. We have a special access that some other bodies cannot gain for certain funds. We have expertise and competence in this area" (Q 1455).

6.69 As well as highlighting the advantages they see of their work, Healthwork UK also identified an obstacle they have encountered in their efforts to develop National Occupational Standards with the CAM professions: "...we have struggled over finance because it is time-consuming, because we have to build consensus so that time is well invested. We need a funded work programme that can last perhaps 3 to 5 years at a time before you begin to see concrete products. Complementary medicine does not appear to us to be a priority from the Department of Health's point of view. It is very hard to help them to put finance aside for this. We have been funded to develop work in public health, in breast cancer, in nursing. The Department of Health is willing and able to apply funds in order to develop National Occupational Standards and their application. It has been much harder for us to achieve funding for CAM. We are quite worried at the moment that we will lose the benefit of the momentum that has been generated" (Q 1146).

6.70 National Occupational Standards are most likely to benefit therapies whose professional organisation is still fragmented and which have not, as yet, managed to agree training standards and objectives. Healthwork UK's support structure and access to funding is also likely to help the smaller CAMs which have fewer resources and less access to funding from their members. The therapies in Group 1 have probably developed beyond a stage where Healthwork can be of maximum help, but for therapies such as those in Group 2 Healthwork UK's clear structures and resources are likely to be beneficial. **We recommend that therapies with a fragmented professional organisation move in this direction and we encourage the Department of Health to support further Healthwork UK's activity in this field; we believe that this would be of long-term benefit to the public.**

Training Conventional Medical Practitioners in CAM

FAMILIARISATION FOR MEDICAL STUDENTS

6.71 Given the increasing popularity of CAM it is important to consider how far medical and other healthcare practitioners should be made aware of the CAM therapies in their training. There are two main reasons why familiarisation is important. First is the belief that doctors should have an understanding of all the health services their patients may be accessing. FIM believe this is particularly important because if doctors do not ask patients about their use of CAM, "there are confounding factors in your delivery of orthodox care...that is bad for the patient" (Q 101). There is an obvious potential for interactions between CAM treatments and conventional medicine. Secondly, medical practitioners (especially general practitioners) are often used by patients as an information source for all health questions. It is therefore necessary, as the Royal College of Physicians told us, for medical students to "have some knowledge of CAM so that they can advise their patients appropriately" (P 190).

6.72 The GMC, whose Education Committee advises medical schools on their curricula, explained that their view towards familiarisation with CAM is positive and that they are actively encouraging medical schools to include this in undergraduate curricula. Professor Graeme Catto, Chairman of the GMC Education Committee, explained: "I think we would want medical students to become familiar with all these techniques, and some, in a sense, are more readily applicable than others, some are already moving into conventional medicine, if you like, and others are far from that. I think the understanding and awareness of what patients may come to young doctors with is helpful in undergraduate medical education" (Q 1037). Professor Catto also said that beyond making sure all medical students had an awareness of CAM there is scope for allowing those undergraduates with a special interest in the area to pursue a deeper understanding of CAM: "Some will want to take that information a stage further and will wish to become involved, through the special study modules, in undertaking some treatments themselves or experiencing, along with patients, what is happening. A further stage then would be through special study modules or related to intercalated degrees. Some may wish to pursue research in these areas".

6.73 Although the GMC believed that familiarisation was important, their evidence confirmed that up until now their guidance in this area has been very vague: "*Tomorrow's Doctors*[44] presently refers only to the need for medical education to recognise that there is a growing demand for treatments that do not conform to the conventional orthodoxies" (P 96). We were pleased to hear that the GMC are now taking a more proactive role. They explained: "*Tomorrow's Doctors* is due to be revised in the

---

[44] The GMC's recommendations on the undergraduate curriculum for medical students, last issued in December 1993.

near future to reflect our view that the universities need to provide some familiarisation with complementary and alternative therapies to students in training".

6.74 We received a wealth of evidence from other witnesses on this matter. The majority (including FIM (Q 1010) and the main professional bodies representing the therapies in our Group 1) have supported the idea that all medical undergraduate courses should include information on CAM.

6.75 The Council of Heads of Medical Schools agree that there is a need for medical education to recognise the growing demand for treatments that do not conform to conventional orthodoxies (Q 245). They gave evidence showing there is enthusiasm for this amongst medical students (Q 243). They stated their position was supportive: "Undoubtedly we perceive interest amongst our undergraduate students in CAM. That is not only in medicine but in other healthcare professions (for those of us who have those within our faculties). The position of the Council of Heads of Medical Schools is that we would be supportive of familiarisation with the philosophy and techniques of CAM in the undergraduate medical curriculum for the prime reason that large numbers of our patients are accessing this form of treatment and it is therefore an important piece of knowledge for undergraduates to have". They proposed that the main scope for programmes of familiarisation lies in two levels: "There should be a small amount of teaching that is for the whole undergraduate corpus, with the ability of those who wish to, to take special study modules and to have more detail on CAM. That is actually quite a common structure amongst United Kingdom medical schools".

6.76 We are aware that there are two approaches familiarisation can take; one is a sympathetic approach to CAM, highlighting its benefits to patients, and the other is an unsympathetic approach highlighting CAM's weaknesses and using it as an example of the dangerous, unproven, unregulated side of healthcare. Both these approaches have been suggested to us. Professor Michael Baum, Professor of Surgery at the Royal Free and University College Hospital, explained that: "As part of the teaching of my medical students I use the claims of complementary and alternative medicine to illustrate the demarcation between science and non-science" (P 243). He assured us he would be outspokenly hostile towards the idea of teaching "alternative medicine" in the undergraduate medical curriculum "other than as an illustration of uncritical thinking" (P 242). However the majority of submissions have suggested that CAM familiarisation should exist so that doctors are aware of their patients' options and can understand why they may be making certain choices. The GMC explained that medical schools teach evidence-based medicine "...so it isn't inappropriate that some schools look at pitfalls related to CAM" (Q 1044). During their regular visits to assess individual medical schools they had found no evidence of any school taking an antagonistic view of CAM.

6.77 We recommend that familiarisation should prepare medical students for dealing with patients who are either accessing CAM or have an interest in doing so. This familiarisation should cover the potential uses of CAM, the procedures involved, their potential benefits and their main weaknesses and dangers.

6.78 During our Inquiry we visited the University of Southampton Medical School and were given a presentation on their familiarisation module: see Appendix 5. We were impressed with the content and approach of the Southampton CAM module and are glad that several other medical schools now offer similar modules. However, overall medical school provision of information on CAM is sketchy. The GMC provided us with some information about the existing provision of CAM familiarisation in some of the other United Kingdom medical schools which were visited during their assessment of Universities' success at implementing the principles set out in the Council's recommendations in *Tomorrow's Doctors* (see Box 8). This showed significant variation in the extent of CAM familiarisation in United Kingdom medical schools.

Box 8

Extracts from Reports of GMC Visits to United Kingdom Medical Schools 1998-99

Teaching of CAM

" *Queen's University, Belfast* — A discussion session on alternative medicine forms part of the Science, Society and Medicine module in phase one.

Birmingham — Since 1993 first year medical students have spent one afternoon of their first term with a complementary therapist. This has allowed each student to observe practitioners from two of the following therapies: homeopathy, acupuncture, aromatherapy, reflexology, hypnotherapy and the Alexander Technique, physiotherapy and osteopathy. Students' enthusiasm for these sessions encouraged the School to offer an SSM [Special Study Module] in complementary medicine in Phase 2. This option has proved very popular and has been over-subscribed since its introduction.

Leeds — The School has developed a computer assisted learning (CAL) package on alternative therapies that will shortly become available. The package provides an introduction to a variety of alternative therapies ranging from herbalism and acupuncture to crystal healing. Self-assessment questions are included so that students can test their knowledge and understanding of those therapies.

  The SSM Co-ordinator told us that demand from students for SSMs in alternative and complementary medicine had allowed the School to establish links with a range of institutions and organisations involved in this aspect of healthcare. Hence contacts have been developed with the Centre for the Study of Traditional Chinese medicine and the North of England Teaching Centre for the Alexander Technique. Titles of SSMs undertaken by students include "Reflexology and Healthcare Today", "Homeopathy – Principles and practice" and "Traditional Chinese medicine – The Back Shu Points".

  We understand the new Health and Illness in Individuals and Populations Integrated Core Unit will include special formal teaching on complementary medicine.

Leicester — The Faculty considers it important that all students should have a good working knowledge of certain complementary and alternative therapies. Accordingly, during Phase I they are familiarised with statutory controlled practices such as osteopathy and chiropractic, and those therapies practised by registered therapists such as acupuncture and hypnotherapy. In the Medical Sociology module consideration is given to the social, cultural and psychological factors which may influence an individual to seek assistance outwith the conventional medical profession.

Newcastle upon Tyne — Some attempts have been made to include this subject within the course. Thus teaching and learning within the Medicine and Society strand promotes an understanding of, and respect for, the health beliefs of individual patients. This programme also considers factors that encourage some people to seek treatments that do not conform to conventional practice. Students are able to undertake SSMs on topics such as "Complementary Medicine" and "The Integration of Complementary Therapies in Medicine into General Practice."

Sheffield — Core teaching in complementary medicine is delivered in Level 5 Lecture Block and Speciality module whilst a Level 1 lecture examines complementary therapies in conjunction with teaching on aspects of neoplasia.

Wales — UWCM acknowledges that little or no teaching is devoted to complementary medicine, though an SSM in this subject is offered....We were told that it was left to the Student Medical Society to organise an event on alternative and complementary remedies available to patients."

Source: General Medical Council (PP 97 – 98).

6.79 We believe that the provision of CAM familiarisation in medical schools is currently too uneven. Some medical schools have well-developed systems for raising CAM awareness in their students, including opportunities for students to observe therapists in action and to attend a small number of lectures as well as the opportunity to take further optional special study modules. On the other hand, other schools have almost no provision for teaching CAM or only briefly mention CAM during lectures on much broader subjects such as Society and Medicine, therefore leaving the task of finding out about CAM to the individual student's initiative. **We recommend that every medical**

school ensures that all their medical undergraduates are exposed to a level of CAM familiarisation that makes them aware of the choices their patients might make. We suggest that all medical schools should consider whether or not to make available optional Special Study Modules in CAM for those students with a particular interest in this area.

POSTGRADUATE FAMILIARISATION FOR DOCTORS

6.80 The drive to raise awareness among medical students about CAM is relatively new, so most qualified medical practitioners will not have touched on this subject in their undergraduate training. In order that existing doctors are aware of this area and can advise their patients on their choices, it has been suggested that CAM familiarisation should be included in the Continuing Professional Development of doctors. This is especially relevant for general practitioners and those working in specialities where they are likely to meet patients accessing CAM disciplines (e.g. epidemiologists, allergists, neurologists). Similar arguments apply to dentists and veterinary surgeons. This view was articulated for us by Ms Julie Stone, a Senior Lecturer in Healthcare, Ethics and Law at the University of Greenwich: "As well as tackling this issue prospectively, it is also necessary to provide familiarisation for those doctors and nurses who did not have access to such initiatives in their training. This knowledge is particularly important for GPs, since they are the health practitioners most likely to provide continuity of care. Postgraduate training and Continuous Professional Development might be a useful point at which to introduce such training" (P 288).

6.81 The GMC told us that "the detail of postgraduate training is...a matter for the Royal Colleges and Faculties and the other competent authorities" (P 96). However, none of the Royal Colleges we have heard from discussed this as an activity they are either encouraging or considering.

6.82 However, the University of Oxford Faculty of Clinical Medicine believe familiarisation in CAM for all doctors is important: "Such training is necessary if doctors are to be able to make use of valuable resources in the community, to give informed advice to patients and to be aware of practice that may be harmful and of where to go for information on possible interactions between pharmaceutical drugs and herbal remedies...It should be incorporated into continuing medical education as well as into medical school training" (P 232).

6.83 The British Dental Homeopathic Association pointed out that most dental patients attend for regular examinations which do not always involve any treatment. This places the dental practitioner with an interest in CAM in an ideal situation to discuss aspects of CAM which are related to dentistry. Advice on nutrition is a good example as oral health is directly related to diet. There are also aspects of osteopathy, acupuncture and homeopathy which can be linked to the maintenance of good dental health.

6.84 In their evidence, the General Dental Council (GDC) (P 75) confirmed that: "A number of factors might lead dentists to consider a more holistic approach to patient care than other professionals." Dentists may be involved in CAM in a number of ways and "there are circumstances in which a dentist might provide treatments which could be described as complementary or alternative which themselves amount to the practice of dentistry. For example, such treatments might be in the areas of pain and anxiety control or oral health education which would be regarded as part of a dentist's normal practice. The Council would have no difficulty in unconventional approaches being employed in such circumstances provided that such approaches conformed with the Council's guidance and the public was not put at risk."

6.85 **We recommend that Royal Colleges and other training authorities in the healthcare field should address the issue of familiarisation with CAM therapies among doctors, dentists and veterinary surgeons by supporting appropriate Continuing Professional Development opportunities.**

TRAINING FOR MEDICAL PRACTITIONERS

6.86 It has been almost universally agreed by our witnesses that the undergraduate medical curriculum should only familiarise students with CAM and not teach them how to practise it. Although several submissions have suggested that CAMs with a proper evidence base should be subsumed into conventional medical practice, this has met with scepticism and occasional frank opposition from the CAM bodies. Therefore, medical practitioners who wish to incorporate CAM therapies into their own practice need to seek specific training in these therapies at a post-graduate level.

6.87 Historically there are many cases of medical practitioners delivering CAM alongside conventional medicine. For example, the Royal London Homeopathic Hospital, which has been part of the NHS since its inception and provides a range of CAM therapies (P 193), has a clinical staff who are "all statutorily-registered health professionals with additional training in Complementary and Alternative Medicine". There is much controversy about whether doctors who want to train in a specific CAM modality need to undertake the same training as a non-medically qualified student of that therapy. Many doctors assert that their previous medical training should allow them to take a much shorter course, as they do not need to learn the basics of anatomy and physiology in the way that non-medically qualified students would. It has also been suggested that the practice of doctors who are delivering an integrated approach is likely to be different from the practice of therapists delivering a complementary or alternative approach, and therefore the emphasis of their training should be different.

6.88 In the Glasgow Homeopathic Hospital (which the Chairman and a member of Sub-Committee I visited in August 2000 – see Appendix 6) medical students are regularly attached to the Homeopathic Hospital on an elective basis. Here they are taught how to use homeopathic remedies of all types but whenever appropriate, and particularly in serious disease, they are trained to use conventional medical treatment. In essence, therefore, they are trained in the practice of integrated medicine.

6.89 FIM has suggested that "it is important that the standards of training and skills of orthodox western medicine practitioners in CAM disciplines is the same as that approved by the appropriate CAM regulatory body" (P 89). We have received evidence from several bodies that have been created to train and support doctors wishing to practise certain CAMs. These bodies tend to have their own training courses, open only to previously qualified healthcare practitioners. There is often limited communication between medically-based and non-medically based CAM bodies. A case in point is the communication between the two homeopathic bodies, the Faculty (see para 5.91) and the Society which represents non-statutory registered homeopathic practitioners.

6.90 The Faculty of Homeopathy accredit postgraduate doctors, dentists, veterinarians and other healthcare professionals who wish to practise homeopathy (P 82). They have developed a specialist examination, and issue qualifications which they say are internationally recognised (P 82). They told us that they are currently working towards a core curriculum which "provides a framework of training requirements for safe and effective homeopathic practice and defines the syllabus for the Faculty's examination. The core curriculum sets out three levels of training for practitioners working in different settings and at different levels of expertise – Introductory, MFHom and Higher Specialist Training. It includes minimum specifications for the subject matter, the time scale of the study and the assessment procedure or "exit criteria" at each level of training" (P 83).

6.91 The Faculty told us that there is very little co-operation between themselves and the Society of Homoeopaths over a core curriculum for training homeopaths. Although the Faculty worked on the development of National Occupational Standards in homeopathy they do not train according to the National Occupational Standards. This is because the Faculty believe the training needs of medically qualified homeopathy students are very different from the training needs of those not medically qualified. There are several reasons for this. The Faculty told us: "In a sense we are not training the same people so a core curriculum for someone starting from scratch to become a homeopath is a completely different training pathway from the core curriculum for a doctor that has done undergraduate training and then postgraduate training" (Q 672). The Faculty's training therefore assumes that people who come to them for training "know what the basic foundation of medical science is and know the structure and function of the body and the mechanisms of disease" (Q 667). The Faculty also believe that medically qualified homeopaths "do not do the same jobs as people who have not had a medical training" (Q 652). "The kind of people who come to a homeopathic hospital will probably of necessity be different from those seeking help in a place where there is no local homeopathic medical provision". Therefore it would make sense for them to have a slightly different training.

6.92 The Society of Homoeopaths agree that "…medical practitioners who have done full medical training do not need to study anatomy, physiology and pathology again" (Q 685). However they assert that "…to achieve full homeopathic competence — and we are talking here of a philosophical shift of perspective on human health and illness — there is a large block of learning and knowledge to be done which is quite different from conventional medical training and, therefore, we would maintain that to be fully competent homeopathically requires full education and training in the same homeopathic knowledge and understanding that the non-medically qualified homeopaths have". We are not convinced that this body of knowledge is derived from a firm evidence base.

6.93 The Faculty and the Society agree that previous medical training negates the need for doctors to complete some parts of the course that would be required of non-medical students. It also seems logical that medically qualified individuals may benefit from teaching specifically on how to integrate their two areas of knowledge, conventional and homeopathic. They also agree on the need for an in-depth understanding of the philosophy and practice of homeopathy itself. However, despite what seems to be considerable common ground, the two bodies have had very little communication over what a curriculum needs to include to provide students with no previous knowledge of homeopathy, with an in-depth understanding of the practice and philosophy of homeopathy. This lack of communication between medical bodies and non-medical bodies providing a specific therapy seems quite common. For example, a similar trend was found between the British Acupuncture Council and their medical counterparts, the British Medical Acupuncture Society.

6.94 As the best use of the same therapy for the benefit of patients is the aim of both the medical and non-medical bodies in each of these cases, it would seem sensible for them to communicate on the best ways of achieving this aim; it may even be sensible to encourage inter-disciplinary learning in some modules.

6.95 The GOsC has managed to find a way of satisfying FIM's idea that the training of medically qualified CAM practitioners should be approved by the appropriate CAM regulatory body. The GOsC approve a college which provides training in osteopathy exclusively for doctors and takes into account their previous training, experience and expertise (p 113). As a well-organised statutory body the GOsC are well-placed to do this, and in fact if doctors want to use osteopathic techniques and call themselves osteopaths they need the approval of the GOsC, so they have an incentive to co-operate. **The General Osteopathic and Chiropractic Councils, and any other regulatory bodies, should develop schemes whereby they accredit certain training courses aimed specifically at doctors and other healthcare professionals, and which are developed in conjunction with them. Similar schemes should be pursued by dentists and veterinary surgeons.**

NURSES, MIDWIVES AND HEALTH VISITORS

6.96 Like doctors and dentists, nurses are often used to provide an information service on healthcare by patients and, therefore, they also need to be aware of the variety of other treatment modalities their patients may be accessing either through CAM practitioners or through health food shops and other outlets. The practice of nursing often incorporates some form of complementary therapy, as a way of relaxing patients or as a part of palliative care. The Royal College of Nursing have suggested that "the therapies that nurses use most often are therapies like reflexology, aromatherapy and massage" (Q 532).

Familiarisation

6.97 We were concerned to hear that, unlike the medical schools, there seems to be little or no evidence of a trend within nursing schools to ensure that student nurses come into contact with the main issues connected to the practice of CAM therapies. This is despite the fact that nurses are probably the most likely of all conventional health practitioners to use CAM techniques in their day-to-day practice. The Royal College of Nursing explained that "At present there is no formal facility for awareness-raising of complementary therapies within the core curriculum. However in many courses it is in fact happening, because it happens naturally in some modules. A module that is focusing on chronic illness will introduce an awareness of complementary therapies, because it is that section of the public who are mostly accessing complementary therapies. Nurses, by virtue of their role of working alongside patients and helping them to gain information, need to understand that this is a choice patients are exercising" (Q 534). Although this suggests that some nurses are made aware of CAM in their training, the Royal College of Nursing were unable to give a clear picture of how common this is because they have not achieved any systematic monitoring of the teaching of CAM within the nursing curriculum.

6.98 The UKCC, the regulatory body responsible for nursing training, said they do not set the curricula for schools of nursing; just the profession's competencies (Q 572). At present an understanding of patients' interest in CAM and its benefits and shortfalls is not considered as a specific competence required of nurses. The nearest they get to issuing such advice is requiring an "understanding of the roles of other practitioners" (Q 570) and they believe this is "equally applicable to the understanding of therapists as it is to the role of the medical practitioner or physiotherapist". But CAM therapists' roles are not explicitly mentioned. It is worth noting that the UKCC does have a role beyond setting competencies in that they support the work of the National Board of Education Providers in determining how their standards will be met (Q 565). They also set the standards for post-registration education.

Training

6.99 We do not have precise figures on the proportion of nurses who practise CAM. The Royal College of Nursing has a Complementary Therapies Forum, which brings together nurses with an interest in CAM. The Forum has a membership of 11,400, which is a rough guide to the number of nurses in the United Kingdom who have expressed an interest in this area of practice (Q 513). Among nurses the popularity of CAM is increasing; this is reflected in the trend in membership of the Forum which was established in 1994, and which in 1997 had a membership of 1600 nation-wide (Q 524). (Its size has more than quintupled in the last 3 years.) However, these figures cannot be used as anything other than a guide to nurses' interest in CAM. Nurses who want to join this group neither have to be practising CAM nor do they have to show any evidence of training in the area; similarly nurses who wish to practise forms of CAM do not have any obligation to become a member of the Forum (QQ 516 & 517).

6.100 There is also no mechanism through which the UKCC can trace how many of their members practise or have received training in CAM therapies. They explained that in the past they "recorded qualifications that would have been recognised by the National Boards" but they found "inherent problems in doing this" and they no longer note any extra qualifications that nurses hold (Q 587). They stated they would "look to other bodies to undertake that, rather than ourselves".

6.101 Having received written and oral evidence from the Royal College of Nursing and the UKCC we are concerned about their passive approach to CAM and the lack of work being undertaken by these bodies in relation to nurses' use of CAM and their training in the awareness of CAM practices. There is a concern that nurses may be exposed to inferior or superficial training programmes and may practise without adequate supervision of this component of their work.

6.102 The Royal College of Nursing's Complementary Therapies Forum has produced some guidelines for nurses wishing to practise CAM. They have produced a leaflet for nurses which sets out questions they should ask before commencing a CAM course; they have also produced a leaflet on the types and levels of courses run in complementary therapy education. However, outside the Forum there seems to be little movement within the Royal College of Nursing or the UKCC towards making sure that all nurses are aware of CAM and that those who practise CAM as a nurse are properly trained to do so. Even for members of the Forum who practise CAM there is no requirement for them to demonstrate completion of training. When asked if nurses in the Forum should logically have had to demonstrate appropriate training, the Royal College of Nursing responded by saying that it was not something they were actively looking into at present (Q 519).

6.103 If neither the Royal College of Nursing nor the UKCC are paying active attention to this field it means there is almost no guidance for nurses who are trained, or want to train in CAM. The Royal College of Nursing did state that it "...seeks to uphold certain standards of practice in specific areas like complementary therapies by engaging in activities like standard setting, trying to promote ideas about the core curriculum when considering the preparation of nurses and by encouraging research activity" (Q 520). However, they had produced a patient information leaflet which encourages patients to ask questions of those people who are offering them complementary therapies.

6.104 The Royal College of Nursing stated that they felt themselves and the UKCC should be responsible for core curricula for nurses wishing to train in this area (Q 537). One of the reasons for this is that the Royal College of Nursing have expressed a belief that the training of nurses in CAM therapies needs to have a different emphasis – one which concentrates on enabling nurses "safely and efficaciously to integrate this therapy in the context of clinical work" (P 118). "The Royal College of Nursing does not aspire to own any core curricula that are developed; although, in the context of complementary therapies, our Forum would seek to have an influence in the development of the core curricula" (Q 537). The Royal College of Nursing's Forum has already begun to do some work in the area of developing curricula for CAM training courses specifically aimed at the needs of nurses: they explained: "I think we need to make it clear that discussions about the development of elements of the core curriculum are at a developmental stage within the Steering Group of the Forum. Those standards are not entirely established" (Q 535).

6.105 The Royal College of Nursing did express concern that there was a variation in the quality of CAM training to which nurses may be exposed: "One of our concerns is that, by advising individual nurses to undertake appropriate training, it is leaving things too much in the open...Until fairly recently, the training that people could access was private and independent, it was of variable standard and often quite expensive, and not focused to the needs of nurses using complementary therapies in clinical practice. This is an area where we feel it appropriate for the Royal College of Nursing to do some work looking at educational standards so we can offer some guidelines to nurses" (Q 531).

Conclusion

6.106 **We recommend that the UKCC work with the Royal College of Nursing to make CAM familiarisation a part of the undergraduate nursing curriculum and a standard competency expected of qualified nurses, so that they are aware of the choices that their patients may make. We would also expect nurses specialising in areas where CAM is especially relevant (such as palliative care) to be made aware of any CAM issues particularly pertinent to that speciality during their postgraduate training.** This is something which the Royal College of Nursing indicated was already beginning (Q 534), a move we find encouraging. We have no expectation that training in the use of any CAM therapy should be a standard part of a nurse's undergraduate training and would therefore expect that nurses who wish to practise CAM therapies would take up such training post-registration. **The Royal College of Nursing and the UKCC, as they do not provide CAM training themselves, should compile a list of courses in CAM that they approve, in order that nurses who wish to practise in this field can obtain guidance on appropriate training.**

CHAPTER 7: RESEARCH AND DEVELOPMENT

7.1 There are many uncertainties surrounding CAM and its practice. In order to respond to these concerns, high-quality research into CAM is vital. Nearly all the evidence we have received has confirmed that research is important in order to ensure that the treatments which the public are accessing are safe, that the efficacy of different therapies can be proved and that their cost-effectiveness can also be established. It is also important to determine why the public are accessing CAM.

7.2 The priority areas for research into each therapy will vary, depending on what, if any, evidence already exists. However, the range of high-quality research activity that has occurred and is occurring in the CAM sphere is minimal.

7.3 Several reasons have been put forward to explain why so little high-quality CAM research is being done. The five most common reasons suggested to us are: a lack of research training across the CAM professions; a lack of research funding available for CAM projects; a poor, almost non-existent, research infrastructure within the CAM sector; a lack of interest in this field of research by conventional scientists who are trained in research methodology; and finally methodological issues, with many CAM practitioners believing that conventional research methods are not suitable tools with which to investigate CAM.

7.4 The three main questions that this chapter will cover are:

- What are the priority areas for research?

- How can the amount of high-quality research be increased?

- How could the outcomes of such research be translated into clinical practice?

Priority Areas For Research

7.5 Important areas for research in the CAM field may be considered to fall into six main categories:

(i)   Research into the effects of each individual therapy; its efficacy, its safety and its cost-effectiveness.

(ii)   Research into the mechanisms of action of each individual therapy, including patterns of response to treatment and research into the placebo effect.

(iii)   Research into the CAM genre itself, including social research into the motivation of those patients seeking CAM and the usage patterns of CAM.

(iv)   Research into new research strategies which are sensitive to the CAM paradigm.

(v)   Research into the efficacy of the diagnostic methods used.

(vi)   Research into the implementation and effects of CAM in specific healthcare settings.

7.6 In the book by Vincent & Furnham[45] referred to in para 3.14 it is suggested that in well-established therapies questions regarding mechanisms of action or the optimum way to deliver treatment may be allowed to dominate research but, in the case of relatively new and untested treatments, questions about safety and efficacy should first be determined.

7.7 To conduct research into the CAM disciplines will require much work and resources, and will therefore be time-consuming. Hence, we recommend that three important questions should be addressed in the following order:

(i)   **To provide a starting point for possible improvements in CAM treatment, to show whether further inquiry would be useful, and to highlight any areas where its application could inform conventional medicine — does the treatment offer therapeutic benefits greater than placebo?**

(ii)   **To protect patients from hazardous practices — is the treatment safe?**

(iii)   **To help patients, doctors and healthcare administrators choose whether or not to adopt the treatment — how does it compare, in medical outcome and cost-effectiveness, with other forms of treatment?**

---

[45]   Vincent, C. & Furnham, A. (1997) *Complementary Medicine: A Research Perspective.* Chichester: Wiley & Sons.

SHOULD SPECIFIC THERAPIES BE PRIORITISED?

7.8 In all medical research a structure of testing exists where treatments with no evidence base are tested first in small-scale studies, and only once some evidence of efficacy has been confirmed are large-scale studies begun. In our opinion those therapies in Group 1 are at a stage where large-scale studies are justifiable because the ground work has already been completed. This is in contrast to the majority of the other CAM therapies where there is little or no objective evidence to support a beneficial effect and as a result small-scale studies are more appropriate. This is the experience of the NCCAM in the USA (see paras 7.84-7.92). Dr Stephen Straus, Director of NCCAM, told us that applications for research funding from those therapies in our Groups 2 and 3 "...are more developmental research applications, what we at the NIH [National Institutes for Health][46] call R-21s, with a neighbourhood of about $100,000 or $125,000. The evidence base is not sufficient to justify what we call an RO-1, which is a full project, which is four times that size. Most of our applications in number are the smaller developmental projects. Most of our funding goes to larger projects within those very few areas where the evidence base is strongest" (Q 1731). We would expect to see a similar pattern in the United Kingdom.

7.9 We believe that those therapies in Group 1 are likely to command the highest proportion of research resources. Those therapies in Groups 2 and 3 will need to build up their respective evidence bases with small preliminary studies before large-scale studies are justifiable.

Research Methods

7.10 In order to address the research questions identified above, it is imperative that research methods are defined that are both sympathetic to the CAM paradigm and rigorous in their design, execution and analysis. We have received a considerable amount of evidence indicating that CAM may have some specific features that makes it less amenable to testing by conventional methods of investigation, most especially the Randomised Controlled Trial (RCT).

7.11 A number of research methods and their applicability to CAM are discussed below.

RANDOMISED CONTROLLED TRIALS (RCTS)

7.12 An RCT is a trial with two defining features. First, control: outcomes for patients in the trial are compared with outcomes for patients in a "control" group who do not receive the treatment. Second, randomness: patients are assigned to the two groups at random, so that any difference in outcome can be attributed solely to the treatment.

7.13 The control population in an RCT can either consist of patients with the same pathology who receive a "dummy" (or placebo) treatment (to test overall efficacy) or a group who receive a comparison treatment to assess whether the therapy under investigation has any advantages in terms of efficacy, safety, cost or other benefits. Where the most important question is whether the effect is psychological, it is crucial to have a placebo control group who believe they are receiving the treatment when in fact they are not. (This is a "blind" trial).

7.14 Much of our evidence states that the RCT is regarded as the most powerful scientific tool for evaluating medical therapies and is accepted as the gold standard in research against which to assess a therapy's efficacy.

7.15 Although many scientists see RCTs as the ultimate analytical tool, RCTs may not fully embrace the CAM paradigm. Some CAM practitioners suggest that RCTs cannot do justice to the individualised, person-centred approach of many CAM therapies.

7.16 FIM explained some of the reasoning behind such claims: "In particular two things are really important in many CAM therapies. Firstly, the idea of standardisation versus individualisation, that actually individualised treatment has a higher value than a standard treatment, and standardising CAM treatments can lead to research outcomes which are not true of the therapy. The second point is that the traditional diagnoses which are used or the hands-on skill...are incredibly important in ensuring a good outcome, and that too has to be taken into account when you look at research" (Q 91).

7.17 The Aromatherapy Organisations Council also explained why they do not believe RCTs are always the appropriate method for CAM research: "It is not necessarily appropriate for all medical and healthcare interventions to be backed by the evidence of controlled clinical trials and by conventional

---

[46] The National Institutes for Health is one of 8 health agencies in the public health service in the USA, which in turn is part of the US Department of Health and Human Services. The NIH is a research organisation, conducting research in its own laboratories and in universities, medical schools, hospitals and research institutes. NCCAM is one office within the NIH.

scientific thinking. As Kleijnen[47] points out: 'the healing process is traditionally in three parts: the self-healing properties of the body; the changes induced by non-specific effects of the therapist and the setting in which the therapy takes place; and specific effects of physical and pharmacological interventions.' In mainstream medicine, the latter usually predominates (but not always) while in complementary medicine it is the second mechanism, and the first process is invariably a factor in both cases. The second may be considered a placebo response and this has made the conducting of randomised controlled trials in aromatherapy difficult" (p 14).

7.18 In March 2000 we visited the Marylebone Health Centre (see Appendix 4) which conducts practice-based research. During our visit, Dr David Peters, a GP and osteopath, discussed the applicability of research to real-life practice. He suggested that although RCTs and meta-analysis of RCTs are valuable, in that they provide certainty about the efficacy of a medication for a particular condition, real-life primary care does not mirror the way illness and treatment are defined in such research. He further explained that many patients do not come to their practitioners with specific, well-defined conditions, but the conditions of entry into most trials eliminates all but the most clear-cut examples of a condition. He suggested that this is especially a problem for CAM as GPs often refer the more complicated patients with chronic, complex conditions to CAM practitioners. Often these patients were not suffering from a single problem; although a particular condition may have been the primary reason for referral, further discussion often unveiled an array of inter-related problems. Thus, the simple definitions of clinical problem and treatment that good RCTs require do not always mirror the complexity of CAM practice.

7.19 Many conventional researchers and medical practitioners have criticised the arguments CAM practitioners use against RCTs, and have suggested that they are just excuses to avoid having to submit a type of therapy to scientific scrutiny. Professor Tom Meade of the Royal Society told us: "I do not see any reason why any of those CAMs cannot be subjected to randomised control trials. There is absolutely nothing different, in principle, between a CAM and a conventional treatment. A lot of ...CAMs have actually already been subjected to randomised control trials" (Q 163). Dr Stephen Straus concurred with Professor Meade's opinion: "The tools of science are such that they can be brought to bear on this field. There is often the prejudice that the tools of science have nothing to add to the field of complementary and alternative medicine. I respectfully disagree with that opinion" (Q 1733).

7.20 Despite accounts that only a few years ago no middle ground could be found between those who rejected RCTs as a research method for CAM and those who advocated them as the only way to prove a therapy's efficacy, we found a growing acceptance from all sides that RCTs had their place but that that place was alongside other research methodologies. Therefore evidence from RCTs must be seen in the context of other evidence from different sources. For example the British Acupuncture Council wrote that: "When researching the evidence for acupuncture, different research questions require different methodologies. To answer questions of efficacy, effectiveness and cost effectiveness, the randomised control trial (RCT) will provide the most vigorous evidence. However where RCTs are too difficult, non-randomised controlled studies, outcome studies and observational studies may provide the best evidence. The variety of research methods range from quantitative to qualitative, and often these two approaches, when appropriately combined, provide triangulation which strengthens the evidence base" (p 28).

7.21 The Academy of Medical Sciences agreed: "...all medical and healthcare interventions should ideally be backed by the evidence of controlled clinical trials and by scientific thinking...evaluation cannot, however, always be achieved by double-blind trial but requires a synthesis of evidence from every reliable source" (p 3).

7.22 It has been suggested that one of the reasons many CAM practitioners are so suspicious of the RCT is because of a widespread perception of the rigidity of such trials and a lack of understanding that their design can be somewhat flexible. For example, not everyone realises that RCTs do not invariably have to be blinded or fully standardised[48] in the way many imagine. Professor Tom Meade described how RCTs can be adapted for different treatments: "Many of them, of course, cannot be double- or single-blind (see para 3.30); the patient and the therapist are both going to know what treatment is being given. There are ways of getting round that. For example, the patient can be asked to go to an assessor who does not know what treatment he or she was having, and in my experience patients enjoy that; they rather like the air of mystery and slight deception that is involved in that. It works very well...I think the point that you make about the amount of treatment varying in some

---

[47] Kleijnen J et al, "Placebo effect in double-blind clinical trials: a review of interactions with medications". *Lancet* 1994. 344,1347.

[48] A common feature of RCTs is that the treatment being administered is given in a standard form to all patients, not allowing for individual difference.

circumstances is not, again, in principle, any different from conventional medicine, and what you may be saying there is that you are testing a package of treatment against some other treatment and you are not necessarily concerned, at that stage, with the dosage effect; you are just wanting to see if patients who have had this treatment, devised according to whatever the therapist thinks is best, will do better than patients who are given another treatment" (Q 163).

7.23 The RCCM confirmed that there is often misunderstanding among proponents of CAM concerning the flexibility of the RCT: "I think from the point of view of CAMs there is, to some extent, a misunderstanding about the nature of the RCT and the fact that perhaps it needs to be blinded, and it does not; it is possible to carry out randomised control trials that are unblinded. There is a question of what is a comparable or useful control because, for example, it is very difficult to find a believable placebo for acupuncture. Various researchers have tried it but it is very difficult to find one. However, what is possible to do is to carry out pragmatic randomised control trials; for example, to randomise patients with a particular problem — chronic back pain for example — into a group where they receive a holistic assessment from a traditional Chinese acupuncturist and then receive individualised care. This group of patients is compared with the best available treatment we have" (Q 129).

7.24 It is clear that, in the treatment of many conditions which are not life-threatening; sequential, longitudinal or cross-over trials (with an intervening 'wash out' period) in which a conventional medicine is given for a period, followed by a CAM therapy, or vice-versa, are powerful and scientifically acceptable methods for assessing the efficacy of a particular treatment. Alternatively, the results of the best-known conventional treatment can be compared with those of a CAM therapy in matched groups of patients.

7.25 Concerns over RCTs distorting a therapy or disguising its efficacy are not the unique concerns of CAM practitioners, there are many potential problems for all therapies when designing an RCT, and these are reviewed in Appendix 1. However, Vincent & Furnham acknowledge that some of these methodological problems are particularly pertinent to CAM research: these are elaborated upon in Box 9.

Box 9

Issues to Consider When Designing RCTs for CAM Therapies

Alternative theoretical frameworks: This is only an issue if two different disciplines have incompatible theories supporting them, which is the case when some of the traditional theories used to explain CAM systems are compared with the scientific basis of conventional medicine. However, Vincent & Furnham point out that this need not matter unduly in clinical trials as long as the CAM practitioners are allowed to practise in the way they see fit and the researchers understand and are tolerant towards the different approach of CAM. They suggest that both sides have to take a 'black box' view of the therapy, by which they mean evaluate it as a package and study the specific ingredients of the package later.

Different diagnostic systems: Patients in controlled trials need to be homogeneous with respect to their disease. In conventional medicine a specific diagnosis is specified but in CAM people are classed in different ways; for example by symptom (meridian imbalances etc). Although both systems may take into account a wide range of information, much of which may overlap, they are unlikely to correspond exactly and the diagnosis will differ. Therefore in clinical trials of CAM an important question to consider is: 'Are the groups going to be homogeneous in terms of a conventional medicine diagnosis or a CAM diagnosis?'

Single-blind or double-blind trials: Some treatments cannot be tested in a double blind format. This is especially true with some physical interventions which require a skilled practitioner who will, of course, know whether they are giving a sham treatment or not. Independent assessment can get over some of the problems of designing trials for such treatments, but independent assessment does not make a trial double-blind. This is also a problem with many conventional medicine treatments including surgery and thus is not an issue unique to CAM.

Individual differences in treatment and responses to treatment: It is integral to many CAM therapies that the patients are treated as individuals. (However, again, this is not a characteristic unique to CAM.) The problem here is that RCTs usually involve the testing of a standard therapy for a standard disease. For some CAM therapies which insist that a treatment strategy should take account of the individual as well as the disease, such an approach would mean that the treatment fell so far short of the optimal therapy that results from such a trial would be irrelevant.

Individual responses to treatment: Some CAM therapists believe the outcome of any treatment results from a unique constellation of factors that are particular to each individual patient. Therefore the controlled trial which obscures individual differences in outcome in favour of group averages and generalisations can seem meaningless to them. Vincent & Furnham observe that trials are a simplification of the clinical situation and that the fundamental questions posed in a controlled trial concern groups of patients and not individuals. Therefore it is important to know what questions RCTs are addressing before criticising their approach or design.

The contributions of the patient and practitioner: The central purpose of a placebo-controlled trial is to separate the influence of the therapy from other factors such as psychological effects of the treatment or the doctor-patient relationship. The very fact that such care is taken to separate out these factors acknowledges the potential influence they have, and yet they are ignored. Vincent & Furnham suggest the lack of research on these factors is regrettable and that CAM practitioners with their emphasis on holism may especially find it so. Ideally, holistic beliefs should be incorporated into research on CAM, although they suggest it is not necessary always to include them for meaningful research to be carried out in this area. Research into patient and practitioner variables is extremely difficult and costly. Psychotherapy researchers have been painfully struggling with these issues for many years. Vincent & Furnham suggest that this means that, however important such issues are, they should not be the first priority for research into CAM.

Source: Vincent, C. & Furnham, A. (1997) Complementary Medicine: A Research Perspective. Chichester: Wiley & Sons.

7.26 Although the design of RCTs for CAM therapies may require very careful attention this is rarely impossible. **We recommend that CAM practitioners and researchers should attempt to build up an evidence base with the same rigour as is required of conventional medicine, using both RCTs and when appropriate other research designs.** How CAM may attract or train researchers with the skill to design such trials, and how funding may be gained to make such trials possible, will be discussed later in this chapter.

QUALITATIVE RESEARCH

7.27 RCTs, sequential studies and comparative studies are all types of quantitative research. Qualitative research employs smaller samples to address more open-ended questions, for example: "what dimensions of x pose what risks, and to what?" Samples of this sort of research are typically too small to be representative, but one important role of qualitative research is to complement quantitative research by identifying and exploring variations of meaning in people's understanding and responses.

7.28 It is also possible to design good quality qualitative research; focus groups have successfully identified end-points which can later be used in an RCT. And rigorously designed questionnaires can provide answers which can be converted into validated quantitative scores. This can deal with issues such as quality of life or can be disease-specific, as in asthma or arthritis.

7.29 Quantitative and qualitative research designs are both important and can reveal different features of a treatment. Qualitative research is important in the early stages of research and has the benefit of being flexible and examining different aspects of the therapeutic intervention than the RCT examines; over the last few years the results from such studies have grown in acceptance and are being used to form part of a therapy's evidence base[49].

7.30 Some other qualitative research designs and their applicability to CAM are reviewed in Box 10.

Box 10

Some Forms of Qualitative Research: Their Advantages and Disadvantages for CAM Research

Case Studies - involve taking a detailed account of the effect of a treatment on an individual or a group. This method is good for studying rare clinical situations, for reporting new information on side effects etc. and for introducing new views and challenging existing theories. Reports from this type of study often provide hypotheses to be followed up in more formal studies. However, case studies cannot prove a hypothesis or generalisation as they are not controlled. Case studies are probably of limited use in CAM where there is already a mass of clinical description and many hypotheses that need testing.

Single Case Designs - an attempt to formalise case studies. For example, different treatments, (perhaps including placebo) may be given in sequence and the effects of each observed and compared with a baseline no-treatment stage. Single case designs have the advantages of being cheap and flexible in approach. They offer different levels of formality and rigour and can incorporate an emphasis on providing the best individually tailored care. Their methodological rigour can equal that of controlled trials. However, single case designs present various problems if treatment has long-term or irreversible effects. They are not suitable for broad questions about applicability of treatments across a range of individuals.

Clinical Audits - progress of patients under treatment is monitored and any adverse effects are noted. There is not usually any comparison group. Clinical audits have been developing strongly in conventional medicine for the last few years. They can be carried out on any aspect of a treatment, and are a good stepping-stone to producing formal studies. Clinical audit does not include a control group, so cannot prove or disprove a hypothesis.

RESEARCH OUTCOME MEASURES

7.31 Research methods are not the only important factor in designing trials; the outcome measures used to measure the effect of a therapy also require consideration. Outcome measures can include both objective and subjective measures. Objective clinical measures include the quantification of physiological indices such as blood pressure or the size of tumour. Subjective measures include symptom scores, patient satisfaction scales and quality of life measures. Traditionally RCTs have concentrated on objective findings although, more recently, patient-centred outcome measures have also been used and some well-established questionnaires have been developed. Nowadays quality of life measures can include measures of pain, physical activity, sleep, energy, emotional reactions and social isolation.

7.32 The research undertaken should identify a single or, at most, two principal outcome measures, and the trial should achieve the appropriate level of significance, (e.g. $p<0.05$ or less). Secondary endpoints can be added. Similarly, composite scores can be used as a primary outcome variable – these would incorporate a number of carefully validated measures, which could be derived by using,

---

[49] See our report *Science and Society,* 3rd Report 1999-2000, HL Paper 38.

for example, principal component analysis, e.g. asthma score, which takes account of symptoms, lung function and treatment requirement.

7.33 During our visit to the Marylebone Health Centre (see Appendix 4), Dr David Peters explained why outcome measures are important and how the Health Centre have tackled the problem of finding measures that can be used in everyday practice. CAM practitioners have utilised a range of questionnaires and interviews. However, many of these instruments required much time and thought from the patients, since the Marylebone Health Centre had decided to opt for a short form of questionnaire that measures only subjective endpoints, which they are now piloting. Their experience has shown that research on appropriate outcome measures that can be used in practice-based research is needed, and this is one of the reasons they are piloting their form.

7.34 The move towards incorporating objective and subjective endpoints into a trial should be reassuring to the CAM practitioner who is concerned with making as broad an assessment as possible of the various changes the treatment has brought about. Vincent & Furnham suggest that there is no reason why measures considered to be especially appropriate for a particular CAM therapy, e.g. changes in the emotional state following homeopathic interventions, should not be recorded and correlated with changes in other measures or indices of clinical change. However, they also suggest that these should not be considered as outcome measures until their reliability and validity have been established.

7.35 The more endpoints used in a study, the higher the chance is of a Type I error. A Type I error is where a change is found on a measure even when, in reality, there has been no improvement. A way of avoiding this is to designate one measure as the primary endpoint and, should this improve, changes on other measures can be examined to confirm any effects of the treatment.

WHICH RESEARCH METHOD TO USE AND WHEN

7.36 It is clear that there are many methods available for conducting research into healthcare interventions. The RCCM, which has 16 years' experience in trying to develop CAM research and getting its results accepted, said: "...there has been a debate about the question of RCTs and their application to the area of complementary and alternative medicine. We think that this debate is unhelpful because, essentially, we need to begin with what are the questions we want to ask and then design the appropriate trial and use the appropriate methodology" (Q 26). We agree. The debate over which methods are applicable to CAM and which are not is probably unhelpful; this dilemma has consumed much energy and has produced strong divisions of opinion in the CAM and conventional worlds. The more useful question is which method is suitable for answering which problem.

7.37 Which method is most appropriate to use will depend on the level of development within the therapy and on the particular questions being researched. This was articulated particularly well by the RCCM: "...the establishment of evidence-based medicine requires evidence from both quantitative and qualitative methodologies. Again, to reiterate, the method is determined by the research question. We would suggest that a range of methodologies should also be employed. Health service researchers are increasingly using qualitative methods. And methods employed in the social sciences should also be employed in the evaluation of CAM, depending on the research question. So we may ask, for example, what it is about complementary medicine that people feel is of benefit to them? Is it a genuine therapeutic relationship or is it [related to] where the needles are placed in acupuncture? They require a different approach. One requires in-depth, qualitative interviews. The questions of how does it affect a patient's quality of life, and how does the therapy affect a patient's physical condition would require a more quantitative approach, such as assessment by using a disability scale or a health status measure. So that the full range of methodologies ought to be applied, depending on the research question"(Q 135).

7.38 FIM produces a useful table showing which methods are suitable for which situations in the Discussion Document *Integrated Healthcare: A Way Forward for the Next Five Years?*

7.39 Mr Michael McIntyre, a trustee of FIM, told us that he believed this controversy over what research methodology should be used was part of the reason why so few CAM practitioners attempted rigorous research: "I think from the CAM side one of the reasons why, perhaps, the amount of research and applications is as low as you say, is that there is a general fear that there is going to be a misunderstanding of the paradigm" (Q 91). It is our hope that, as more CAM practitioners are trained in research methods, and are made aware of the different types of research design; and as more conventional scientific investigators become aware of the intricacies of CAM research, this 'general fear' will be overcome.

Expertise on Grant-Awarding Boards

7.40 Given some of the complexities in designing trials for CAM, it has been suggested by several of our witnesses that there is a particular need for members of grant-awarding bodies to understand the specific problems facing CAM research in order to be able to make a fair and well-informed judgement on the importance and quality of a proposal for funding. The British College of Naturopathy and Osteopathy (P 31) also suggest that to counteract the feeling that many Research Councils do not give CAM proposals a fair chance, funding bodies should recruit CAM members with the appropriate research qualifications to help determine the validity of protocols.

7.41 We asked some of the main funding bodies whether they thought that there was a need for them to appoint specialists in this area on to their boards. The MRC told us: "We do have boards that can judge the proposal. The Health Services Research Board contains a wide range of people, not necessarily practising complementary and alternative medicine but people who understand research methodologies, research questions and can judge whether those questions are answerable using the methodologies that individuals can formulate. I think we do have the people who can judge those things" (Q 1087).

7.42 The Wellcome Trust also defended the composition of their panels: "The panel system that we have within the Trust is a very strong one and is based on peer review. If within the panel there is a lack of expertise we have the option to co-opt an expert to deal with the particular application. If there was a complex CAM application it could then be dealt with by bringing a specialist on to the panel. The panel itself would make the decision, taking account of that expert's advice. The Trust goes to great lengths to get proper peer review. We employ 90 scientific officers to send out all of the bids we receive for peer review. We believe that that is important. To date, we have received 163 CAM applications. The indications are that 37 per cent of those have been funded. That proportion is higher than we would expect for our more orthodox applications, which routinely is about 30 per cent" (Q 1132).

7.43 We asked the Association of Medical Research Charities (AMRC) whether they thought their member charities' boards had the relevant expertise. They too felt that their current provisions were fine and that there was no need to change their system to give CAM proposals a fairer wind: "As an Association we are committed to the use of peer review and believe that that is the best way for charities to make judgements about the best use of their funding. But peer review is quite a flexible system and it should not be applied in a rigid way. The AMRC's guidelines accept that there are certain areas in which one may need a different review process, but the key principle is that there should be an internal and external process of peer review. Where specific expertise is not available on the panel we insist that those charities must seek it externally and choose external referees in an open way. We provide support and advice for charities in identifying external referees. One possibility is for AMRC to draw up a list of potential CAM external referees, although charities do not indicate that they have any difficulty in identifying referees through the normal process of literature researches, networks and various other ways. We also advise charities to go overseas so that questions about the status of organisations and the networks in which particular individuals feature are diminished" (Q 1190).

7.44 The AMRC went on to describe one particular initiative by one of their member charities to aid CAM applications. "The Arthritis Research Campaign is about to introduce a mentoring process of peer review for CAM applications. Even if they are of lower standard initially, applications will be picked up by a member of the panel and taken through with guidance by specialists to try to raise the standard of specific applications. Only very large charities with significant staff can take on that mentoring role. It is an example of how the peer review process can be used to give feedback and to raise the standard of an application so that it can come back again. I do not believe that there is anything inherently wrong with the peer review system for CAM research. I hear criticisms of peer review from every speciality" (Q 1190).

7.45 Overall it would seem that the majority of funding bodies are now willing to ensure that CAM research proposals are reviewed by well-informed individuals. **To achieve equity with more conventional proposals, we recommend that research funding agencies should build up a database of appropriately trained individuals who understand CAM practice. The research funding agencies could then use these individuals as members of selection panels and committees or as external referees as appropriate.**

Environment and Infrastructure for Research

7.46 There are currently a variety of different environments in which CAM research is conducted in the United Kingdom. These vary from university-based research departments which operate as part of well established medical school research departments, to projects based within charities and in clinical practice either in hospitals or in primary care.

7.47 During the course of our Inquiry we visited three different research environments. Two of these were university-based research departments. The first was the Department of Complementary Medicine at the University of Exeter, which is based within a school of postgraduate medicine and supports the United Kingdom's only CAM Chair. The second was based within a school of medicine — the Complementary Medicine Research Unit of the School of Medicine at the University of Southampton. The third research environment we visited was an NHS clinical practice — the Marylebone Health Centre, an NHS inner-London GP practice which offers CAM therapies alongside conventional care and which supports practice-based research. (See Appendices 3, 4 and 5.)

7.48 We heard much evidence in favour of establishing and supporting a few centres of excellence in CAM research, such as those at Exeter and Southampton, as opposed to spreading funds and resources across many disparate projects. FIM's discussion document *Integrated Healthcare*: *A Way Forward for the Next Five Years?* suggests that "it would seem appropriate to concentrate resources on establishing a number of research centres linked with higher education institutes with the capacity to conduct high-quality research into CAM".

7.49 This is the approach of NCCAM in the USA. Dr Stephen Straus, the Director of NCCAM, told us: "The eleven centres we fund to date are really intended, in part, to draw those CAM practitioners and experts into the fold of a larger research enterprise within an established community. Out of the many hundreds of institutions in the United States we are creating foci within only one dozen or so and we hope that we will see leaders in the coming years" (Q 1734).

7.50 The Wellcome Trust also supported the idea of centres of excellence and suggested these should be encouraged to develop from existing centres of research excellence to avoid the delays in generating high-quality CAM research. Dr Howard Scarffe of the Wellcome Trust told us: "I had an opportunity to visit one of the clinical research facilities that we fund at a large university teaching hospital. I was excited that another venture was to be undertaken by the Trust with Government under the Joint Infrastructure Fund. Within 25 yards of that clinical research facility the Wellcome Trust is to fund research laboratories…It is very exciting that attached to a large university teaching hospital campus is a clinical research facility in which all researchers can work together. Adjacent to that is a purpose-built world-class laboratory. We are also funding a director of the clinical research facility so that he or she can give full attention to getting it off the ground. It struck me…that if we had good facilities and researchers we could begin to graft on other bits, of which complementary medicine might be one. If one began to build capacity from the ground level there would be a lag of between 10 and 15 years to train people up to a high level. Therefore, there is a need for a system whereby the research can be grafted on to what is already there and use made of the present expertise" (Q 1141).

7.51 Although concentrating funding in a few centres of excellence has many advantages this does not mean there is no place for smaller practice-based research projects. As previously noted, there are many different ways that CAM research can be conducted and large-scale RCTs are probably best conducted in centres of excellence; qualitative research may be ideal for practice-based research.

7.52 At the Marylebone Health Centre (see Appendix 4) we heard from Dr Sue Morrison, one of the senior partners. Dr Morrison explained that as a practice they favoured rigorous clinical audit and have used such data to develop a manual of integrated care for other practices to use. However, she described some limitations to their data. For instance, some patients self-select the Marylebone Health Centre in order to have access to CAM and therefore wider information is needed from across the Primary Care Group on what patients want from their healthcare and, within this, the role of CAM.

7.53 Dr David Peters at the Marylebone Health Centre described how research has the capacity to serve both practitioners' and patients' needs. For example, audit ensures quality assurance, research through qualitative methods increases understanding of the patients' experience, action research promotes service and professional development and case studies illustrate best practice models. In this way practice-based research promotes quality and understanding.

7.54 We received written evidence from the University of Westminster Centre for Community Care and Primary Health (CCCPH) (P 234) which is also run by Dr David Peters. As well as awarding degrees in various CAM therapies and conducting research in this area, the Centre runs a clinic. They explained the advantages of an educational and research department having links straight into a clinic: "The Polyclinic is creating unparalleled educational and research opportunities where students in the BSc and Masters' programmes will gain practical clinical and research experience under the supervision of some of the United Kingdom's most experienced and best-qualified practitioners…As a multi-disciplinary complementary therapy teaching, research and service delivery resource, the

Polyclinic will be unique in Europe and the CCCPH are looking to develop national and international education and research partnerships" (P 235).

7.55 As we discussed in Chapter 5, several of the newer universities now offer CAM courses. The aspiration is that these courses will help establish more university-based CAM research. The BMA told us that they expected these newer universities to be "important players in the field of research in much the same way that medical faculties have a role within medical research" (Q 354). They added: "The question is whether those faculties have sufficient experience yet in devising research protocols, and clearly it is important that they work together to share that experience. Again we believe that organisations such as the Medical Research Council should also be able to offer their help and support in these early stages in the devising of trials and protocols" (Q 354).

7.56 We also asked the CVCP whether they thought the newer universities had the infrastructure to support good quality research. They told us they believed that they did: "The quality assurance regime which the universities operate through the Quality Assurance Agency, which is a tough, self-regulatory regime, would expect every university to consider those issues in respect of any programme: it would expect to ascertain that each university has the appropriate infrastructure which, in certain types of programme, would have to include a research base for mounting a programme. The inspections which are done by the Quality Assurance Agency would certainly cover those areas" (Q 281). They also told us that the regulatory mechanism is there to ensure that no university is left thinking that they will supported if they are mounting programmes without the necessary infrastructure (Q 281).

7.57 From the evidence we have received it is clear that there has been a change of attitude of a few higher education institutions towards CAM as a legitimate subject for both quantitative and qualitative research. However, the small base and fragmentation from which this research will have to be conducted would seem to be a major barrier to progress. **We recommend that universities and other higher education institutions provide the basis for a more robust research infrastructure in which CAM and conventional research and practice can take place side-by-side and can benefit from interaction and greater mutual understanding.** A preferred model would involve centres of excellence committed to establishing a wider framework of conventional scientists, social scientists and CAM practitioners. These would provide a basis for enhancing research into CAM while ensuring it was of high quality, addressed relevant questions and was integrated with conventional methodology. Advantages would be gained by facilitating multi-disciplinary research with access to medical, psychological, social-scientific and pharmaceutical clinical trials. **We recommend that a small number of such centres of excellence, in or linked to medical schools, be established with the support of research funding agencies including the Research Councils, the Department of Health, Higher Education Funding Councils and the charitable sector.**

RESEARCH EDUCATION

7.58 An interest in science or clinical research is not at present a requirement for all CAM training courses, although some schools are introducing courses on research and research projects. Our evidence has helped us construct a picture of the attitude of CAM practitioners towards research. There is an increasing number of CAM practitioners who believe research is important and are willing to put their time and effort into it, but very few appear to have sufficient knowledge or skills in research to advance their interest.

7.59 In the USA one of the main ways that NCCAM is hoping to improve the capacity to conduct CAM research is to improve the education in research methodology of those involved in CAM. This is done through the funding of career development awards at various levels. Dr Stephen Straus, the Director of NCCAM told us: "I believe that those awards need to be to individuals who will be mentored by outstanding scientists and have a protracted period of tutelage, a minimum of three years and ideally five years, to cultivate their skills as an independent investigator" (Q 1734).

7.60 We talked to various United Kingdom funding bodies about the prospect of them awarding research fellowships directed towards students with an interest in CAM in order to invest in the long-term future of CAM research development.

7.61 Although the Government were eager to highlight the importance of education and training in research, they do not currently have a route for supporting research fellowships in this specific area. When we asked Professor Sir John Pattison, Director of NHS Research & Development, how he saw such fellowships being supported, he told us: "I think we have a track record of building capacity in areas of orthodox medicine. Primary care is the first example we embarked upon. In collaboration with the Chief Medical Officer we are about to embark upon similar research training fellowships and career scientist awards in public health...If one simply took those as models for how one would start to build capacity in any area of research to health and health services, then that would be the way to do it" (Q 1869).

7.62 Dr Howard Scarffe of the Wellcome Trust told us he saw the Trust as having a role in supporting programmes which provide training and support in research methodology in the area of CAM. However, the Wellcome Trust's current policy towards awarding PhD studentships is likely to disadvantage CAM applications as applicants without conventional medical or scientific training are likely to be excluded from applying. Dr Scarffe told us: "At present our policy is oriented towards people with medical or scientific qualifications" (Q 1161).

7.63 The Department of Health told us that they saw encouraging research training as one of the best ways of improving the research capacity within CAM: "The approach of the R&D programmes to this and, indeed, all of medicine has been very much to encourage access to training as well as access to research funding. That is provided through a number of mechanisms, including training in research design, training and methodology regionally and centrally. There is a groundswell of movement towards a higher standard of education for researchers. I see that move on the part of the professionals as key to increasing the volume and quality of research that is done" (Q 15).

7.64 The MRC also support research training. They told us: "...our fellowship schemes include fellowships in subjects allied to medicine, and people in complementary medicine are open to apply for fellowships — as they are in...Health Services Research" (Q 1087).

7.65 As well as attracting mainstream experts to investigate CAM, the MRC also explained they have mechanisms for advising people from all areas who need help in designing trials: "...the new MRC Unit on clinical trials, which has a division without portfolio - which is already giving advice to people in trials in areas where traditionally we have been rather weak. That includes advice to particular individuals on how to conduct a trial on complementary medicine" (Q 1085).

7.66 Many CAM university degree courses now include research modules and this is likely to catalyse a change in CAM practitioners' attitudes to research and the need for evidence-based practice. FIM summed up this change: "...we have a lot of university degree courses and very good levels of training being brought into being...and...in nearly every case there is a research module. It does require undergraduates of CAM to...undertake at least some training in research so that the culture of research is encouraged...and that is a very important feature of the education of CAM practitioners — so that we have a common language between researchers in the orthodox field and those in the CAM field" (Q 91).

7.67 Thus, while there currently exist some research training opportunities available to CAM practitioners, none of these is specifically directed towards CAM and very few, if any, of these fellowships have been taken by individuals conversant with the practice of CAM. There may be two principal reasons for this. Firstly, if a practitioner has received no basic education in research methodology he or she is unlikely to seek specialised research training; this is why we hope that CAM regulatory bodies will include research methods in their core curricula (as discussed in Chapter 6) and why the new university courses in CAM represent a promising development. Secondly, the reason why few CAM people take up research training opportunities may well be that they do not know about them. **Bodies such as the Departments of Health, the Research Councils and the Wellcome Trust should help to promote a research culture in CAM by ensuring that the CAM sector is aware of the training opportunities they offer. The Department of Health should exercise a co-ordinating role. Limited funds should be specifically aimed at training CAM practitioners in research methods. As many CAM practitioners work in the private sector and cannot afford to train in research, we recommend that a number of university-based academic posts, offering time for research and teaching, should be established.**

ATTRACTING MAINSTREAM INVESTIGATORS

7.68 Training CAM practitioners in research will undoubtedly increase research activity in this area, but this will take time. An alternative approach would be to attract mainstream investigators into CAM research. This has several advantages: firstly, there would be no time-lag; secondly, such individuals would bring their experience and expertise to this difficult area; and thirdly, such a development could establish links between the conventional and complementary sectors, increasing mutual understanding.

7.69 NCCAM in the United States has been successful in attracting mainstream investigators to address some of the research priorities. The Center's Director, Dr Stephen Straus, who himself is an eminent and successful mainstream scientist, told us: "The more immediately successful route is to seduce your best scientists to join the enterprise, by funding them to work in areas they are already expert in and, perhaps, inherently interested in as well. Our largest funding has been going to our best mainstream investigators. We also need to bring complementary and alternative medicine experts and practitioners into this. That is hard because — except for some very isolated aspects within the chiropractic and the acupuncture communities in the United States and some experts in botanicals — there is not a research tradition in those communities" (Q 1734).

7.70 The MRC were also enthusiastic about this approach to kick-starting CAM research. Professor Sir George Radda, Chief Executive of the MRC, told us: "The first and, perhaps, most critical thing is that we do have a number of very distinguished people who are, if you like, part of the Medical Research Council who actually take complementary medicine seriously and who are interested in taking it forward in some way. Professor Tom Meade, of course, has done one of the pioneering studies on back pain and chiropractic. We have a number of other scientists who have served on various committees that are concerned with complementary medicine...I think people are interested in making sure that not only do we contribute to the debate but that we will be able to do something serious about making sure that the way complementary medicine is used is effective and well-researched" (QQ 1085 & 1086).

7.71 Sir George also explained how the MRC may be able to aid such associations: "We do have the mechanism to encourage those sorts of collaborations. For example we have had, for three years, the co-operative grant system where we encourage people to tackle individual major problems in a way that different scientists can contribute different aspects to that. It would be perfectly reasonable, for example in a co-operative on asthma, to include a component grant application from somebody who wants to develop a study on the use of complementary medicine in asthma, and it would actually then be done in the context of what else is going on in the way of research in asthma, rather than as an isolated project which, perhaps, would not stand up in the long run" (Q 1087).

Research Funding Sources

7.72 Funding for healthcare research, including CAM, is available from a variety of sources. These include:

(i)   the Government

(ii)   the medical research charities

(iii)   commercial and industrial sources

7.73 We have considered the prospects for CAM research under each of these options in turn.

THE GOVERNMENT

7.74 In their written evidence the Department of Health explained that the Government supports health research in the United Kingdom through a number of routes outlined in Box 11. The Government were keen to emphasis that CAM projects may stand a better chance of funding if they come in under areas that the Department of Health are making a priority. Professor Sir John Pattison, Director of NHS Research & Development, told us: "I think the Government has set some challenging priorities for R&D and granted some extra resources for that – but it is in specific areas such as cancer, mental health, cardiovascular disease and coronary heart disease in particular, and the elderly and children. It would be in those areas that we would particularly welcome and look at proposals for complementary and alternative approaches. Just as an example, we are about to fund a study of reflexology in patients after surgery for early breast cancer. I think that reflects that there are opportunities for CAM professionals and practitioners to come through with proposals to get funded through our systems" (Q 1866).

Box 11

Government Funding Options

—*Medical Research Council.*

—*Department of Health 'Policy Research Programme' (PRP)* – This aims to provide a knowledge base for health services policy. PRP has supported two CAM research projects through the Sheffield University Medical Research Unit.

—*NHS Research and Development Levy* – Money is allocated following evaluation of bids competing against national criteria. In April 1998 £360 million was allocated in the form of three-year funding arrangements. One CAM bid was successful in April 1998 and received funding of £61,650 for its first year.

—*NHS Executive Research and Development Programme* – Work is commissioned directly from Universities on behalf of the NHS. There are three main national programmes run under this budget: the Health Technology Assessment Programme, the New and Emerging Applications of Technology Programme and the Service and Delivery Organisation Programme.

—*Methodology Programme* – Supports all the other programmes by commissioning research into methodology. Several projects of relevance to CAM research (although not directed solely at CAM research) have emerged from this programme.

—*Research funded by NHS Regions* – Regions can identify their own priorities 12 CAM projects have been successful in obtaining funding through this route.

—*Higher Education Funding Councils grants to universities* – For those researchers based in academic institutions.

Source: Department of Health written evidence (P 101)

THE MEDICAL RESEARCH CHARITIES

7.75 The structure of the medical research charities means that CAM is often in a difficult position to compete for their funds. The AMRC point out that "Most medical charities spend the greater part of their money on understanding the mechanisms of disease, not efficacy. Usually, efficacy is a smaller part of the work of medical charities" (Q 1198). They also explained that as most medical charities are relatively small and only focus on one or two specific disease areas, it is relatively difficult for them to participate in large-scale, non-disease-specific research funding, which is the usual nature of CAM research. "In this field very few medical charities are general charities. Very little CAM research would be disease-specific. If most of the smaller charities are disease-specific the research simply does not fit"(Q 1176). One important exception is the Wellcome Trust which, like the MRC, will fund research in any area of medical science.

7.76 Currently the AMRC has no plans for special initiatives into CAM: "We are feeling our way as to the role in CAM that might be played by AMRC. AMRC does not have any of its own funding for research. Therefore, the Association is a facilitator in helping charities to spend their money as effectively and in as targeted a way as they can. What we will do is probably take the first step by establishing a special interest group within AMRC to look at CAM research...For it to work it is very important for AMRC to work with the professional body concerned...Partnership with the professional body is important and must be developed in CAMs" (Q 1175).

7.77 As another example of the perceived need for more research into CAM accessed by their patients, the Arthritis Research Campaign has developed an initiative to encourage more CAM proposals with an appropriate assessment mechanism to ensure these will address relevant questions with high-quality proposals.

7.78 There are some small charities dedicated to CAM but, as the RCCM told us, they rarely have the resources to fund research: "Smaller charities - and we are one of them - in the health arena almost always focus not on research but on support for clinics or disadvantaged groups" (Q 117).

COMMERCIAL AND INDUSTRIAL COMPANIES

7.79 For much of conventional medicine it is the large pharmaceutical companies which fund clinical trials. However, in CAM there is very little industry-based research. This is mainly because many CAM remedies are natural products which cannot be patented, and hence companies that research them cannot guarantee that they will benefit financially from the research. Dr Stephen Straus, Director of NCCAM in the USA, explained the situation he has encountered with industry: "There is woefully little investment on the part of private industry. They have yet to discern that there is a financial advantage for them to do so…I am attempting to encourage them to help invest in studies of the effectiveness of their products as well. By and large, they are not doing so" (Q 1712).

7.80 The Wellcome Trust pointed out that, despite the lack of patents on CAM products, industry does make substantial profits in this area, and Wellcome's view is that some of this should be ploughed back into research and development. We agree. They told us: "One interesting matter referred to by Dr Mike Dexter, the Director of the Trust, in his introduction to a workshop on CAM run by the Trust, was an article in *The Times* just prior to that meeting on 2 March which suggested that £500 million in the United Kingdom was spent on complementary health products. The pharmaceutical industry would spend some 25 to 28 per cent of the money from sales of conventional medicines on research and development. Therefore, one might think that in CAM health products perhaps £150 million a year could be spent on research and development" (Q 1136). With no patent protection available for most of CAM such figures may not be easily obtainable in this area. Nevertheless it should be noted that a Research and Development budget of 5% of commercial turnover on CAM products, if this is indeed £500m per annum, would yield £25m per annum. They also suggested that a new regulatory framework for CAM products might encourage industry to invest in the area: "Legislation such as regulations governing pharmaceutical products would help to promote research into CAM products. Of the three major funders of biomedical research in the United Kingdom in conventional medicine, the pharmaceutical industry is by far the biggest supporter. The Government and charities come lower down the list. We believe that perhaps a look at the legislation and regulation of these products may also have a safety spin-off but also release money for further research and development" (Q 1136).

7.81 **We therefore recommend that companies producing products used in CAM should invest more heavily in research and development.**

PUMP-PRIMING AND RING-FENCING

7.82 One method of kick-starting research into CAM is to pump-prime or ring-fence research funds. Ring-fenced funds are funds specifically directed into a defined area of research, and are awarded to applications from that area without having to compete with applications submitted from other areas. Pump-priming differs from ring-fencing in that funds are only dedicated to the area for a limited period of time to help develop the infrastructure needed to underpin substantial high-quality research which will then attract more substantial funds.

7.83 The issue of ring-fencing and pump-priming is controversial and the views of our witnesses on this subject were polarised. Several witnesses suggested that without ring-fencing or pump-priming, the research infrastructure for CAM will remain poor, and that bias and lack of expertise (see 5.38 above) on behalf of research proposal referees will continue to prevent grants being awarded in the area, with the result that CAM research will never be adequately supported. However the alternative view, articulated by several other witnesses, is that ring-fencing and pump-priming are inherently unfair, and that research proposals should all be considered on merit. It is further argued that, by designating funds for a specific area, many problems may arise largely due to an imperative to spend funds on research irrespective of its quality or importance.

The Lessons of NCCAM

7.84 Research funds have been ring-fenced for CAM in other countries, most notably in the USA, where NCCAM received $70 million this year and expects to receive funding of between $80 and $100 million next year (Q 1712). This, however, represents less than 5% of the total budget of the NIH. The history and experience of NCCAM confirms the possible beneficial effects of ring-fencing of research funds in this area.

7.85 NCCAM was only established in 1999: it was preceded by the Office of Alternative Medicine which was set up in 1992. In the first few years of the Office of Alternative Medicine, funding was much lower than that which NCCAM receives and the success of that office in generating good quality research was perceived to be poor. For example, the Academy of Medical Sciences told us that the office had run into serious problems, as many of its research grants resulted in papers being written that were not published or were not published in reputable peer-reviewed journals; hence, they argue against ring-fencing. We asked Dr Stephen Straus to comment on these failures and on the history of his Center: "The first ring-fenced funding, as it were, for complementary and alternative medicine began in 1992, with an allocation of $2m to the then Office of Alternative Medicine, which was in the office of the Director of the NIH. The attempt was for that small office to attempt to leverage those funds and convince the other Institutes to increase their support. The office also funded a number of very small projects. The average funding for each of those projects was about £20,000 (i.e. $30,000), which is somewhat less than one-tenth of the usual size of an NIH grant. It was not surprising that that amount of funding yielded very little in the way of powerful science" (Q 1718).

7.86 However, he said that now NCCAM's increased funding and experience means that they are able to conduct reputable trials: "I would say the best opportunity we have had is to have the independent authority to issue grants at the standing NIH level. We believe we are investing in the kind of research now that will be in the best journals. I would be stunned if our study of *St John's Wort*, that has just recently completed enrolment, would not be accepted in, perhaps, the British Medical Journal. Frankly, I would be, personally, gravely disappointed if we do not do far better" (Q 1718).

7.87 Dr Straus went on to elaborate on how NCCAM had managed to improve the quality of its research. "There were approximately 40 small grants given from the Office of Alternative Medicine in its first few years. With the creation of NCCAM in early 1999 several things were done. First of all, we have invested in creating research capacity, by funding eleven centres to date. Two of the centres fund botanical research. We are funding nine centres around different diseases and conditions. Each of those centres is funded with $1.5 million a year for five years. We are developing research capacity through those centres. We have called for and are now beginning to fund, for the first time, major research, training and curriculum programmes in institutions around the United States. We are attempting to inspire young individuals who seek careers in research to enter the research area within complementary and alternative medicine by working under the mentorship of outstanding investigators. We are funding approximately 80 grant applications at this point, averaging about $250,000 to $300,000 each. We are funding five large, multi-centre, placebo-controlled, randomised clinical trials. Our first large studies will not be completed for little under a year. Our small developmental projects are now entering their second year. It is still premature to know what our funding has bought. We have encouraged very good people to join our enterprise" (Q 1719).

7.88 Dr Straus acknowledged that ring-fenced funding is always a controversial matter in science: "At the NIH we believe, as you do here in the MRC and other leading research funding authorities, the best science is investigator-initiated application submitted by the best individuals in pursuit of the best ideas" (Q 1712).

7.89 However, he also told us that "The funding at the NIH, which this year totals nearly $18 billion is, in many regards, entirely ring-fenced in that it is allocated and apportioned to institutes on the basis of the perceived public health needs in those areas...Our funding is ring-fenced in the broadest sense. It is in pursuit of a broad field and a broad set of ideas" (Q 1712).

7.90 Dr Straus explained the advantages of ring-fenced funding at NCCAM, including the fact that the money does not have to be used just to fund particular projects but can be used to strengthen the research infrastructure: "We have the ability within NCCAM to target our resources in pursuit of the best opportunities. We are building a research infrastructure and capacity by funding centres. These are things the other Institutes would not tend to do for complementary and alternative medicine. We are funding research training and curriculum development from pre-doctoral through career awards. We could invest in areas that are still scientifically unformed but which are matters that are still very much in the public interest. As you know, homeopathy is less well-established in the United States than it is here. We do not have the equivalent of the NHS homeopathy hospitals. We have the ability to fund research. Through the peer review process, which manages all of our grants and applications, we attempt to select the best. It is ring-fenced, in a sense, but it is in response to public need" (Q 1712).

7.91 He went on to elaborate upon how NCCAM decide which applications to fund and explained that scientific merit is considered as one of several important factors: "[Judgements are] made on scientific grounds, while being conscious of the imperatives that we have. Let me explain further. The applications that are received are peer-reviewed, as all applications are to the NIH. They are scored accordingly. It is my responsibility to meet with an advisory council three times a year to review the applications and the scores they receive. My council can, in their best judgement, not change the scoring, but they could say "although this had an average score we feel this is a very important area, or a less important area" (Q 1716). In other words, they can prioritise to an extent.

7.92 Dr Straus also explained how he believed the NIH managed to avoid ring-fencing distorting the overall priorities of health research: "Over the past decades public advocacy has grown in strength and impact...Every important condition has its advocacy organisations that are calling for support for their work. To some extent, there is an equalisation through the process. The US Congress responds to calls on the part of the public, but also to our testimony and our best judgements as scientists as to where the opportunities are greatest and investments are most likely to prove profitable. There is a danger that if that was the only mechanism by which large funding decisions would be made, then there would be a distortion. Fortunately, that is not the only mechanism. Even within that mechanism those are general guidelines. The NIH is still able to fund the very best peer review research" (Q 1714).

Attitude of UK Research Funding Bodies

7.93 The issue of ring-fenced funds has been raised as a means of boosting CAM funding in the United Kingdom in several submissions. Professor Edzard Ernst, who holds the CAM Chair at Exeter University (P 229), points out that ring-fencing has been very successful in other countries (e.g. Germany and the USA) and could be encouraged by the NHS, the MRC, Primary Care Groups and Trusts, and industry. However our discussions with the main research funding institutions in the United Kingdom reveal little enthusiasm for ring-fenced funding for CAM research.

7.94 The MRC do not believe that they should ring-fence funds for CAM. They told us that they intend to continue to judge CAM grant applications by merit in competition with all other grant applications: "The MRC believes that there is no justification for a different approach to research into complementary therapies compared to conventional therapies. At present, there is generally insufficient evidence to prioritise within or between evaluations of conventional and complementary therapies. In the absence of well-developed research proposals, we therefore consider the case for increased research funding for CAM has not been made. Nevertheless, the MRC will continue to welcome applications for support to evaluate complementary therapies. These will be judged case-by-case on their own merits, in competition with other calls on MRC's funds" (P 139).

7.95 One of the MRC's main arguments against ring-fencing funds for CAM is that, given that one of the main problems within CAM is the poor quality of CAM research proposals, ring-fencing might lead only to more poor quality research. They suggest that there are better alternatives to ring-fencing to improve CAM research: "Throwing money at bad science does not help anybody. So I am not for ring-fencing. Whether one should have an initiative, or if encouragement is sufficient, I do not know. In view of what we hear, that the research capacity is not there yet, it seems to me that you need to start training and you need to start getting people who themselves would like to do research in complementary medicine to acquire good research training. That is, train people in statistical aspects of medicine and train people in how to evaluate evidence and so on. Then we could, perhaps, build on that (Q 1095). It is a chicken and egg situation and I believe that people have to come first before you can do the research. You need to target individuals who can do research and say to them: 'this looks now an important enough issue: could you put together a proposal?' That is one way of bringing in the practitioners of complementary medicine as part of such a proposal. That they can, through an individual like Professor Meade, learn how to do this sort of research" (Q 1097).

7.96 Although the MRC were against ring-fencing, they were not against prioritising certain research areas: "...If you say that there are some very, very urgent problems which require proper scientific study that lead to a long-term solution, I am sure we would be very willing to consider it. If it is a matter of comparing one treatment with another, that is more a Health Department issue. With that proviso, there is no reason why we could not respond if there was a real demand from the medical, scientific, or whatever, community for something like that" (Q 1099).

7.97 The Department of Health told us that they also believe that CAM research must be considered on the same basis as conventional research: "The Government views research into CAM in the same light as that into all other branches of medical practice" (P 113).

7.98 The Department of Health fund research through several different programmes and organisational structures (as reviewed in Box 11) and some of these mechanisms allow the setting of priorities: "Priorities for R&D are set from time to time to take account of Ministerial priorities and priorities for health and social care, and CAM research is considered as part of this" (P 114). They did describe one time-limited funding programme that had resulted in some CAM research: "The National Cancer Programme contained a specific priority on the comparison of cost-effectiveness of different psychosocial interventions, including CAM therapies. One CAM project was funded: a randomised controlled study of the effects of reflexology on mood, adjustment, quality of life and patient satisfaction" (P 113). There is also scope for prioritisation within local NHS R&D budgets: "Regional R&D budgets are intended to allow Regions to identify and support local priorities and build research capacity. As part of a Commissioned Research Initiative, South West Region issued a specific call for proposals in May 1996 into: Which specific CAM therapies are effective for which conditions? Which specific conditions may benefit from CAM? What are the resource and other consequences on the NHS where CAM is not provided or used? As a result of this call, two projects were funded: a project – now complete – to evaluate the effectiveness of acupuncture in defined aspects of stroke recovery (£179,903), and a multi-centre study of acupuncture for tension headaches (£22,169)" (P 113).

7.99 As discussed in paragraph 6.81 Professor Sir John Pattison, Director of NHS Research & Development, and Yvette Cooper MP, Parliamentary Under Secretary of State for Public Health, both encouraged CAM proposals to try to come in under current NHS initiatives, such as those prioritising cancer research. However, despite these limited initiatives, the general position of the Department of Health is not one that favours ring-fencing or pump-priming: "Within the NHS R&D programme there has been relatively little ring-fencing in any area. The arguments against ring-fencing are robust. I believe that it would imply a dual standard and at the end of the day there must be research that is robust enough to give clear answers, By relaxing the standards of rigour it is too easy to make research investments that do not pay off" (Q 5).

7.100 We also talked to non-governmental bodies about their attitudes to dedicated funding. The Wellcome Trust told us that, despite their recent conference on CAM and their belief that it is an important area: "CAM research is not ring-fenced, and it is probably our policy not to do that" (Q 1104). Although in the past Wellcome did ring-fence, they explained that "we now go for open competition and try to reduce the number of schemes that we fund by bringing them together so that all who apply have an equal opportunity" (Q 1104). The Trust do have some directly-managed initiatives, for example on genomes, but they saw this as an unlikely prospect for CAM (Q 1168).

7.101 The AMRC explained why they did not believe that ring-fencing was an option for medical charities: "We would resist the idea of any medical research charity being perhaps forced to ring-fence money for a particular speciality. In a way, that money is already ring-fenced for specialities or diseases. That is not a comment on the need or not for Government to ring-fence; it is a fact of life for charities" (Q 1194).

7.102 It is our opinion that despite the Department of Health and the MRC's reservations about dedicating funding, something must be done to build up the research capacity in CAM; otherwise the poor state of research and development in this area will continue. The lessons of NCCAM in the USA show that, if funds are there, experienced researchers will apply for them, and with sufficient investment high-quality CAM research can be achieved. NCCAM's annual budget is about $68.4m: this is 0.4% of the total budget of the NIH. Without dedicated funds, CAM will struggle to attract high-quality researchers and it will be hard to build the infrastructure for the research that needs to be done in this area to protect the public. In our opinion it will not be long before CAM research will be able to compete against other bids for funds in a way that it cannot currently do. **We recommend that the NHS R&D directorate and the MRC should pump-prime this area with dedicated research funding in order to create a few centres of excellence for conducting CAM research, integrated with research into conventional healthcare. This will also help to promote research leadership and an evaluative research culture in CAM. Such funds should support research training fellowships and a limited number of high-quality research projects. This initiative should be sufficient to attract high-quality researchers and to enable get them both to carry out large-scale studies and to continue to train CAM researchers in this area within a multi-disciplinary environment. We believe ten years would be sufficient for the pump-priming initiative as, for example, in the case of some MRC programme grants and various training and career development awards available in conventional medicine. The Association of Medical Research Charities may also like to follow this example.**

Co-ordinating the Development of CAM Research

7.103 The discussions in this chapter show that there are many issues to take into account when considering how to increase research into CAM. Several of our witnesses have suggested the need for a co-ordinating body to promote research in this area. For example Dr Howard Scarffe of the Wellcome Trust felt it may be sensible to have an "over-arching organisation to co-ordinate research strategy" (Q 1136). He went on to suggest that "the Foundation for Integrated Medicine may possibly be an appropriate organisation to assume that role" (Q 1136).

7.104 A body of this sort could take on various roles to aid CAM research:

(i)   To act as an advice centre on where to gain research funding;

(ii)   To advertise funding programmes;

(iii)   To act as an information centre on research training opportunities and to advertise specific opportunities in this area;

(iv)   To advise on drafting grant applications;

(v)   To disseminate research findings and co-ordinate research strategies.

7.105 FIM told us: "I think our central role at the Foundation in relation to research is very much encouraging others to do it. That might involve the Government, it might involve the Wellcome Trust; it certainly does involve the research charities which are responsible for nearly £500 million of research, so we see our role as very much one of influencing and helping. Part of that may involve us directly funding some research; we do have a small research programme ourselves but it needs to be seen within that wider context" (Q 93). FIM are currently drafting a national strategy for CAM research.

7.106 The RCCM also believe that there is a need for a national strategy for CAM research. "Given the public and professional interest in complementary and alternative medicine, a co-ordinated strategy supported by public funds requires careful consideration and debate (Q114)... In the absence of a comparable R&D infrastructure, CAMs do not have a national strategy, so any research will be carried out in isolation, will be ad hoc and will not address key priorities. So we feel that a national strategy is required" (Q 118). They believe that this national strategy should be "developed and co-ordinated by a body that is independent of but accountable to Government. It should have relevant and appropriate multi-disciplinary representation from both the CAM field and the conventional field, and appropriate representation from health service researchers, and there is a current debate in NHS R&D around a lack of good health service researchers. It should be chaired, or led, by someone who is impartial and not immersed in a particular tradition, and it should establish priorities for CAM research, perhaps through a consensus approach drawing on the multi-disciplinary field. It should commission, fund and monitor CAM research including the quality of the research that it is commissioning" (Q 352).

7.107 To maintain impartiality and fairness, but not at the expense of quality, FIM is in a particularly strong position to take on these tasks with resourcing from the Government and possibly the charitable sector. Joint research between different grant-awarding bodies is gaining acceptance in the United Kingdom and therefore we see no reason why, with appropriate safeguards and accountability in place, the Research Councils and the Department of Health could not drive forward CAM research by operating in this way, rather than by simply awarding individual grants. There already exist examples of such mechanisms in the concordat that the MRC and the Department of Health have developed for joint working, and the joint initiatives between the United Kingdom Government and the Wellcome Trust in the Joint Infrastructure Fund and Joint Proposal Funding Initiative.

CHAPTER 8: INFORMATION

8.1 The popularity of CAM raises important questions in terms of information provision and validation. For a patient or a doctor wishing to find out more about a CAM therapy, information will be required to answer the following questions: What is involved in the treatment? What conditions do its advocates claim it can treat? What is the evidence to support these claims? What might be the side-effects? Whose views can I trust? For patients, two further questions are likely to be: What does my doctor think about it? and What conventional medical treatment should I compare it to? Doctors are likely to ask: What is the consensus medical view?

8.2 If once these questions are answered the patient or doctor decides they would like to consult or refer to a CAM practitioner, another set of questions arises: Is the treatment available on the NHS? How much does it cost privately? Where are the local practitioners? Which ones are well-qualified and proficient?

8.3 Healthcare administrators may wish to have other types of information, such as the latest publications on delivery systems for CAM, or figures covering the latest trends in CAM use.

8.4 Although in many circumstances needs for, and uses of information by, doctors and patients overlap, there are particular issues which are more relevant to one group than the other, and in this chapter we address separately information provision for doctors and healthcare professionals, and for patients.

8.5 Towards the end of our Inquiry a conference was organised on the subject of information sources in CAM[50], and we have tried to include some of the items which were raised there in this chapter. However, the quantity of information on healthcare, including CAM, which is now available, is immense and increasing rapidly, and we have not been able to address all the various sources in depth.

8.6 FIM told us that the current state of information provision in the CAM area was patchy and disorganised. "There are some useful sources of information for patients and doctors regarding complementary and alternative therapies, but these are disparate, reflecting the fact that much of CAM is provided outside the NHS" (Q 87).

Information for Healthcare Professionals

8.7 Doctors need access to good quality information concerning CAM. This is especially true for GPs, nurses and pharmacists, all of whom are often used as health information resources by the general public. Healthcare professionals need information not only to answer patients' queries about their treatment options, but also to understand what their patients are talking about if they discuss their use of other therapies.

8.8 We heard from Dr Simon Fradd, a GP, giving evidence for the BMA, about the problems doctors currently face due to the variable quality of information available about CAM. He told us: "There are real problems about quality control of the data that we are getting. At the moment we are still at the stage of being able only to discuss the concept of referring to an alternative practitioner rather than having an evidence base that says 'in back pain you should take this step if you have found these features'. My own committee at the BMA, the General Practitioners' Committee (GPC), published guidance in July last year for items that should be taken into consideration when a colleague is thinking of either delegating or referring to an alternative practitioner. What that indicates is that any of this information as it develops needs to be shared between the various professions" (Q 361).

8.9 In Chapter 6 we discussed the need for medical, nursing and other health-care education to incorporate CAM familiarisation courses into their training curricula. This is the first important step towards making sure that healthcare professionals are well-informed about CAM. However, information delivery needs to continue beyond the years of undergraduate education so that doctors can keep up with advances in the field and can, with changes in patients' demands, expand their knowledge of areas especially relevant to their practice.

8.10 The BMA also believe that the representatives of individual therapies should be in charge of collating information for each such discipline. They told us that CAM professional bodies should work with others and look at examples of best practice in the field to guide them. "They should then work with others and that might be in other specialities of CAM or it might be people in conventional medicine, and it might well be patient groups and others, to try and put together information both for the public and for conventionally trained doctors. There are a lot of examples where guidelines have

---

[50]   On 31 October 2000 by the Foundation for Integrated Medicine and the British Library.

been issued by organisations including the Medical Royal Colleges, increasingly they have been from the National Institute for Clinical Excellence, on clinical areas..." (Q 357).

8.11 It is also important that conventional healthcare individuals and organisations can identify and contact the lead professional bodies in CAM. Guidance is needed in this area, especially in the case of the more fragmented therapies which have several representative bodies. It would be helpful if each health authority had available a CAM information pack giving contact details of the different professional bodies, and a directory of CAM services available in the area as they do for dentists. This idea was supported by FIM (Q 85).

8.12 A positive move has recently been taken in this direction as the Department of Health, together with the NHS Executive and the National Association of Primary Care Groups, have produced an information pack about CAM for primary care groups. This was distributed to all PCGs and is available on the NHS website. This pack identifies the main bodies representing the therapies most commonly used in primary care. It is discussed in depth in the next chapter. However, although this pack addresses some of GPs' information needs in relation to CAM, it is a national document and so does not address the need for local directories of CAM services, nor does it cover all the main CAM disciplines.

THE DISSEMINATION OF RESEARCH FINDINGS

8.13 New advances in CAM need to be well documented and easy to identify. Hence, the dissemination of research findings is an important factor in information provision for conventional healthcare professionals.

8.14 Currently the results of CAM research are published in many different journals. Some of these are highly reputable conventional medical journals, but others are less well-known and the published papers are less rigorously peer-reviewed. Much research in CAM is published in journals dedicated to CAM which have small circulation figures and are unlikely to come to the attention of GPs and conventional medical scientists. Indeed, we have heard some evidence that there is a bias within the larger, better-accepted journals against publishing CAM research, even when it is of good quality. If this is true it must evidently militate against the results of CAM research being properly disseminated.

8.15 Professor Edzard Ernst told us about bias in publications during our visit to the Department of Complementary Medicine at Exeter University. One survey the Department conducted involved submitting two almost identical papers to CAM and conventional medical journals. The two papers both reported fictional results of a randomised controlled trial that showed positive results, one for a CAM therapy, the other for a conventional therapy. They found that the paper based on a conventional treatment was more likely to be accepted for publication by a conventional medical journal than was the paper which reported identical clinical outcomes from a CAM treatment.

8.16 The fact that CAM research papers are published in such a variety of journals, both conventional and complementary, combined with the difficulty CAM research has in being accepted into the more widely read conventional journals, means that the dissemination of research findings in the CAM area faces some special difficulties that need to be addressed. Given the diversity of journals in which CAM research may be published, sources such as the British Library are useful for those who would like to survey all of the published studies of CAM. Indeed, the British Library maintain databases on healthcare information, including AMED (the Allied and Complementary Medicine Database) which collects together CAM articles from about 500 journals from 1985 onwards.

8.17 The NHS Centre for Reviews and Dissemination at the University of York (p 444) commissions and supports experts to undertake specific systematic research reviews in areas of priority to the NHS. They suggest that support should be given to efforts to synthesise all the best CAM research into systematic reviews, such as those found in the database on the Cochrane Library CD ROM, *Clinical Evidence* (produced by the *British Medical Journal*) and *Best Evidence*. They also told us that although they have not, to date, undertaken systematic reviews in the area of CAM, "given our experience and expertise, if we were asked to do such reviews we would be able to undertake them given adequate time and resources" (p 444).

8.18 The UK Cochrane Centre[51] has been mentioned as a useful resource by several of our witnesses. The Department of Health suggested that the Cochrane Centre's application of "rigorous

---

[51] The Cochrane Centre was opened in 1992. It supports the preparation of systematic reviews of randomised controlled trials of health technologies. Several other countries (USA, Canada, Australia, Denmark, Italy, Germany) have opened similar centres to form the "Cochrane Collaboration". Archie Cochrane was an epidemiologist working in Wales in the 1970s, a powerful supporter of randomised controlled trials and author of *Effectiveness and Efficiency*, an influential monograph.

systematic approaches" to reviewing research offers "models that others can use and adapt to suit different fields of reviewing". They also told us that currently the Cochrane Database of Systematic Reviews contains some CAM reviews, although those they could identify were a very limited number (P 114).

8.19 The most comprehensive collection of CAM research references in the United Kingdom is that held by the Research Council for Complementary Medicine (RCCM)[52]. They told us: "The need for a reliable information resource that is accessible to both health professionals and users of complementary medicine alike is central to the work of the RCCM. The RCCM, using mainly charitable donations, has developed the Centralised Information Service for Complementary Medicine (CISCOM), a database of over 65,000 references to research published world-wide since the early 1960s" (P 181). RCCM explained that such a database has uses above and beyond simply finding out about the results of trials into the efficacy of different therapies. "Those planning research have used CISCOM to look at approaches used by previous researchers. Drawing on data from resources world-wide, CISCOM offers a one-stop shop for users. The challenge in the coming years is to offer information to consumers that is readable, based on research evidence, evaluated, and readily updated" (P 181).

8.20 The RCCM also told us that they felt that there could be useful input in this area from NHS bodies: "Emerging NHS strategies in the information field are welcome. The National Institute for Clinical Excellence, the Centre for Health Information Quality and the electronic National Library for Health should include the need to gather data as to the safety, effectiveness or adverse effects of CAM. The RCCM is happy to be involved at every stage of this process" (P 181).

8.21 **We recommend that the NHS Centre for Reviews and Dissemination be invited to work with the RCCM, the UK Cochrane Centre, and the British Library to develop a comprehensive information source with the help of the CISCOM database, in order to provide comprehensive and publicly available information sources on CAM research; and that resources be made available to enable these organisations to do so.**

Information for Patients

8.22 The Department of Health told us: "We believe that it is very important that consumers have access to adequate and appropriate information" (Q 54), and all our witnesses have agreed. The Consumers' Association articulated how important this is: "Our Consumers' Association remit is to lobby on behalf of consumers to improve services and goods. One of our core principles is that people must be able to make informed decisions (about healthcare in this case) and that is about having access to accessible, accurate and complete information" (Q 838). They had done some work themselves towards filling the information gap in this area. "Through our magazines (particularly through *HealthWhich?* for example) over the last year we have run a series of articles on different kinds of complementary therapies, and provided readers with the information that is available in relation to their effectiveness, and given readers advice if they want to seek this therapy on the best way to get information and contacts" (Q 838).

8.23 Most of our witnesses have agreed that the best information sources whereby patients can obtain information about individual therapies are the various professional organisations which represent each therapy. This was the view of the Department of Health: "The Government see it as the primary role of governing bodies of professional groups to provide information to the public. They are best placed to provide advice on the type of treatment to be provided, its appropriateness, how it will be delivered and what the patient may expect from it" (Q 60).

8.24 One problem in this regard, however, is that a statutory regulatory body may be unable, within their legal terms of reference, to give professional advice, other than being able to say whether or not an individual is a registered practitioner. Hence, colleges of the relevant practitioners and/or professional associations could prove to be more appropriate reference sources. The different responsibilities of the GMC, the Medical Royal Colleges and the BMA may serve as examples. The important question here is how will the patients know which body or bodies to contact?

8.25 The Consumers' Association expressed concern about the professional regulatory bodies or professional colleges or associations being used as the main information resource regarding each therapy: "One of our concerns…is about bodies that are more trade associations fulfilling the main role as being providers of information to the public about therapies. That would concern us in a way that we feel it perhaps is not the most appropriate arrangement to be in place. What we would look for

---

[52] The RCCM is a charitable organisation, which should not be confused with Government research councils PPARC, EPSRC, NERC, MRC, ESRC.

are a number of different approaches. First of all, we think it would be very appropriate and necessary for a body that holds the register of practitioners to provide patients or consumers with information about whether individual practitioners are registered and in good standing should they make a request — that is very appropriate. We also think that at some point it may be agreed there is a need for a separate body" (Q 849).

8.26 In any case, while representative bodies are useful sources of factual information - what the treatment involves, where local practitioners are, and what different qualifications mean - independent guidance about the general effectiveness or otherwise of the treatment might best be sought elsewhere. The obvious place to turn is to a GP, but unless he or she is unusually well-informed, this is likely only to shift the problem of having no information from the patient to their doctor.

8.27 Clearly, it would be helpful if there were some point of reference where views on efficacy could be collected together. It would be desirable to have indicated whose views were represented, and the type of evidence each view was based on (clinical trials, anecdotes, or no evidence). Patients and doctors could then survey the various forms of advice available and choose the recommendations of whichever group they trusted most.

8.28 Another problem arises if patients are not sure which therapy is best for their condition and therefore do not know who to contact. In such circumstances, as the Federation of Clinical Shiatsu Practitioners explained, the process of contacting each individual therapy organisation "becomes confusing and costly when trying to identify which therapy would be most beneficial. A central source, furnished with the contact numbers of the said regulatory bodies, would be the most effective system. It may well be worth considering the use of an established system such as NHS Direct" (P 85). The British Holistic Medicine Association explained that currently there is no overarching CAM information source: "For information on…extent of service provision, applicability of different CAM therapies to different conditions…the BHMA [British Holistic Medical Association] and other organisations – FIM, RCCM, Natural Medicines Society (NMS), etc. — are working to fill the current gap" (P 40).

8.29 The Consumers' Association told us that the current information resources within the NHS may be able to provide information in this area and that their role is not being maximised: "We would look for things like the Centre for Health Information Quality which has a remit to provide information to patients. We would want them to include within their work information about complementary therapies. This is NHS-funded and is specifically about providing information to patients. We could see a role for NHS Direct to provide information along with other organisations, for example the College of Health. Rather than taking the leap from here to saying we think there needs to be another body set up, I think our starting point would be that we would like to see the existing processes and centres for information provision used better to provide consumers with information" (Q 849). They went on: "For example, when the NHS published its information strategy two years ago one of the things they proposed, which we strongly endorsed, was the creation of exactly that, as part of the electronic National Health Library, a site where patients could go to look at information that had met very specific standards set by that agency. We see no reason why information about complementary therapy should not also be part of that. At some point there is need for the recognition of a body specifically with responsibility for complementary therapy and information about them to be set up. At this point we are not confident that these processes already in place are being used to the maximum that they should be" (Q 852).

8.30 The potential role of NHS Direct as a source of information on CAM has been brought up by several witnesses. The Department of Health were willing to consider it as a possibility. They told us: "One of the matters on which the Department is actively seeking views in the context of the role of NHS Direct is how information on healthcare can be made available, and one area is alternative medicine" (Q 59).

8.31 **We see the NHS as the natural home in the United Kingdom for reliable, non-promotional information on all types of healthcare; providing such a home is particularly important for CAM, where the diversity of opinion and organisations make it almost impossible for individuals to gain an overview. Consequently we support these plans and urge that they be carried out in the very near future. We recommend that the information should contain not only contact details of the relevant bodies, and a list of NHS provision of CAM in each local area, but also some guidance to help patients (and their doctors) evaluate different CAM therapies.**

8.32 One existing information source that the Department of Health suggested could be amended to provide an information source for patients is the information pack on CAM they produced earlier this year for PCGs (Primary Care Groups) and doctors. Yvette Cooper MP, Parliamentary Under Secretary of State for Public Health told us this was a line she was interested in exploring: "That is quite a helpful guide to people in terms of what evidence there is available about different kinds of therapies. And what organisations exist to regulate them as well. That is the kind of information people want to have" (Q 1886).

8.33 Even if the NHS did not wish to come to a single definitive judgement on the efficacy of each therapy, there seems to be great value in providing, in a neutral forum, a collection of the views of the principal bodies with relevant knowledge.

Media Coverage of CAM

8.34 Other information resources about CAM are the press and other public media. Many of our witnesses, including the Department of Health, recognised that this was one of the main sources of information in this area. "We see a lot of it in the media and newspapers. From time to time newspapers carry articles on complementary medicine, very often in features in women's magazines and consumer programmes" (Q 54).

8.35 A recent study by Professor Edzard Ernst sought to determine the frequency and tone of newspaper reporting on medical topics in the United Kingdom and Germany. The study examined four UK broadsheet newspapers and four German newspapers on eight randomly chosen working days in 1999 and analysed the content of all the medical articles. A total of 256 newspaper articles were evaluated and, with particular reference to CAM, four articles were found in the German papers and 26 in the UK newspapers. All of those in the UK newspapers were positive in their attitude towards CAM, whereas of the four German articles only one took a positive attitude to CAM. On the other hand, the UK newspapers' attitudes towards conventional medicine were more critical than the German. Professor Ernst, communicating these findings to the *British Medical Journal,* commented "…in view of the fact that both healthcare professionals and the general public gain their knowledge of complementary medicine predominantly from the media, these findings may be important."

8.36 FIM told us: "The public is increasingly exposed to information on CAM treatment and therapies as newspapers and magazines give ever-increasing editorial coverage on the subject. Some, but by no means all, of this is well informed. It is therefore essential to ensure that the public has access to high-quality information, which is regularly updated" (Q 87).

8.37 FIM's view of the media's coverage of CAM was somewhat cautious: "What we do is very much to welcome the greater interest and I think this type of information is illustrative of that greater interest. But some of the information is questionable and unless there is some central way of kite-marking or some authoritative place where people can go and get information, there will be a mix of what is available locally, and it varies. I think it is important, as my colleagues were mentioning, that there is information in a form which is helpful for people who are looking for and wanting to know about different treatments" (Q 86).

8.38 FIM continued by pointing out that "Newspapers and television companies are in the business of selling their newspapers and programmes and that very often is what determines the story. This weekend, for example, there has been the continuing saga of *St John's Wort* published in a number of Sunday papers, and one of the stories I saw I helped the journalist with. I gave a lot of information to that journalist and none of it appeared in the story simply because it did not suit the very scaremongering angle this particular story took, which is unfortunate because there is a genuine story there. There are definite issues around the use of this herb and we need to be aware of them, but in some of the stories the driving need is to sell the newspaper and unfortunately reasoned debate does not always sell newspapers" (Q 88).

8.39 We asked the Consumers' Association what they thought of media coverage of CAM. They told us: "I think we can look at this in a positive way…People are getting a lot more information these days. The public are becoming more discerning. There is definitely a role for individual consumers in making their own choice about whether they follow information or not. Having said that, it is important that information is examined carefully. We have a rigorous process of verification, checking with external specialists and experts before any information is provided to the public. In the media short reports appear on papers that have been recently published; however there should be an impression of the general state of research in an area as well as the single exciting new finding" (Q 850). In our report on *Science and Society* we looked at the issue of science reporting in the media, and recommended that the media uphold a series of recommendations suggested by the Royal Society, which included guidelines on accuracy, credibility, balance, legitimacy, responsibility and how to report in cases of uncertainty. We again recommend these guidelines to all health journalists. However, in *Science and Society* we also concluded that science cannot expect special treatment from the media, and it will be necessary for bodies to work with the media as it is. Once individual professions are organised under a single professional body, and an evidence base has been established, it will be easier for the media to know where to get advice and for each body to develop a relationship with journalists to build confidence.

The Internet

8.40 Health information is arguably the most common topic searched for on the Internet, and there is a bewildering number of sites with information in this area. As far as CAM is concerned, the BCMA told us there has been a "proliferation of sites" (Q 603/5).

8.41 As an information source, the Internet has significant merits: low-cost distribution of material worldwide available 24 hours a day. It also has disadvantages: the information available is of a highly variable quality, reputable and disreputable information sources can be hard to distinguish, information is often unattributed or out-of-date.

8.42 We asked several witnesses if they could think of any way of controlling the quality of CAM information on the Internet. Most acknowledged that currently there is no way of controlling what people put on their sites, but several witnesses suggested that kite-marking sites may be a viable option. For example. FIM told us: "The idea of kite-marking seems absolutely essential and the concept of peer review of course is normal practice in conventional medicine and beginning to be normal practice in CAM. If there were information resources put out on the Internet and web sites, it would be good if they were kite-marked and peer reviewed, and I think many people in the CAM area would welcome that process" (Q 83).

8.43 The Natural Medicines Society believed that instead of trying to attempt to control information "it is more a case of setting the quality ourselves and even beyond that being able to place a kite-mark on other sites and say 'these seem to us to be dependable', because there is this great proliferation now of sites both of a CAM nature and of a general medical nature" (Q 1571).

8.44 However, several witnesses told us that kite-marking on the Internet is a flawed process open to abuse. For example, the Patients' Association had already experienced problems with people using their logo without their knowledge: "Our logo has been used as a kite-mark by an organisation that we have no connection with at all. It was only by pure chance that we found that, so we are actually very suspicious of any success with any of this, frankly, on the Internet. When you discover that, how do you police it, particularly with health in general? To do the searches you would have to have somebody employed full-time in every organisation checking up on this to see if their particular logo or kite-mark is being used. The Internet is a real problem" (Q 916).

8.45 The Consumers' Association told us of an alternative to kite marking which they are piloting called a web trader scheme, which looks at the standards that some sites are operating. However this scheme is not particularly looking at CAM sites and they acknowledge that it "is only a step in the right direction. We do not have a solution as to who should fund this" (Q 851).

8.46 The Consumers' Association view (para 8.39) that people are becoming more discerning in judging the information that comes their way may start to reduce the widely held concerns about the way people regard Internet information. In the meantime, while it may be impossible to prevent people accessing incorrect healthcare information via the Internet, it is certainly possible to make it easier to connect to accredited, reliable sources. There is clearly a great deal of activity in this area, and it has not proved possible for us to investigate it all in depth. However, sites such as the OMNI health information gateway, which appears to offer promising initiatives (www.omni.ac.uk), provide searchable access to Internet resources that have been quality-evaluated: it is funded by the United Kingdom's Higher Education Funding Councils through the Joint Information Systems Committee, and the pilot project by the British Library and the Research Discovery Network for a healthcare portal site, which will include CAM. We were pleased to hear of the recent conference on CAM information, organised jointly by FIM and the British Library, and we would welcome any developments which would bring together the expertise of these two organisations in creating portals or gateways for CAM information on the Internet.

8.47 However, initiatives by organisations such as those above may only address part of the problem. Although systems designed for academic researchers, or by organisations whose main constituency is already relatively well-informed on CAM, may be used by the wider community, most people in the United Kingdom would turn first to the NHS for information on healthcare. In terms of web-based information, this consideration means that any information resources on CAM provided by NHS Direct Online or the NHS's electronic National Library for Health will be extremely important in guiding people's choices in seeking or avoiding CAM treatments. Although CAM may not be high on NHS Direct Online's list of priorities as it develops and widens the information it supplies, it should be remembered that in the absence of widely recognised, non-promotional, and reliable information on the web, people may be relying on low quality or misleading sources which they have found by chance. Since many if not most patients will also be turning to their GPs or specialists for advice on CAM, NHS involvement in this area is inevitable. It would make good sense for this to be backed by sound web-based information, especially at a time when doctors might not yet feel competent to give well-informed advice.

8.48 **We are aware that the National electronic Health Library and NHS Direct Online plan to have information available about CAM in the future; we support these plans and recommend that they are carried forward.**

Advertising CAM

8.49 One way for CAM practitioners to disseminate information about their therapy is through advertisements. There are, of course, restrictions on the claims that can be made in advertisements. The Trade Descriptions Act 1968 and the Consumer Protection Act 1987, enforced by local authority Trading Standards officers, apply to professions, including complementary therapists, which make claims for the goods and services they sell. There is also legislation relating to specific illnesses and medical conditions – for example cancer and venereal disease – which prohibits non-medically qualified individuals from purporting to cure them or even, in some cases, to treat them (P 104).

8.50 Some of our witnesses have expressed concern that some CAM advertisements may be extending unacceptably the boundaries of acceptable advertising, and that there may be a need for tighter policing. For example, the Consumers' Association wrote that: "The British Code of Advertising and Sales Promotion states that advertising by complementary therapists should not discourage people from having essential medical treatment; that medicines or therapies for serious or prolonged ailments should not be advertised; and that advertised products or therapies should not claim to be guaranteed to work or be absolutely safe or free from side-effects. It is important that this continues to be enforced in the area of complementary medicine — a small but significant number of practitioners continue to make claims for therapies which cannot be substantiated" (P 66). They recommend that "Information and advertising material should not make claims for complementary therapies that cannot be substantiated by research. All bodies producing such information should be aware of and comply with this requirement" (P 66). In our opinion, while CAM therapists should not discourage patients from seeking medical treatment, nor give guarantees of a cure, we can see no obvious reason why they should be prevented from offering help with chronic (prolonged) conditions, by methods which are substantially free from side effects, since this is precisely where they appear to be helping some patients at present.

8.51 The Consumers' Association went on to elaborate that "In terms of advertising in health generally, not just complementary therapies but health in a broader sense, we have some concerns about the appropriateness of using advertising as a means of conveying information" (Q 860). Such arguments apply equally to advertisements of non-prescription medicines and remedies and not just those relating to CAM.

8.52 Advertising can come in many forms and the Consumers' Association told us that their concerns extended to the leaflets that many CAM associations and practitioners put in consulting rooms which, they told us, are covered by the rules of the ASA (Q 861). They told us that: "The evidence base is really important there. These leaflets should not be written by PR people, they should be written by people who know what the evidence base is for a claim. We have no problem with information from evidence-based leaflets" (Q 862).

8.53 We received written evidence from the Advertising Standards Authority (ASA) which "supervises the advertising industry's system of self-regulation; promoting and enforcing the highest standards in all non-broadcast advertisements" (p 389). They highlighted the parts of the British Codes of Advertising and Sales Promotion most relevant to the regulation of CAM advertising. These are:

- Medical and scientific claims about health and beauty products should be backed by trials conducted, where appropriate, on people.

- Advertisers should not discourage people from having essential treatment; medical advice is needed for serious or prolonged problems and advertisers should not offer medicines or therapies for them.

- References to the relief of symptoms or the superficial signs of ageing are only acceptable if they are substantiated. Unqualified claims such as "cure" or "rejuvenate" are generally not acceptable.

- Advertisers should not use unfamiliar scientific words for common conditions" (p 390).

8.54 The ASA gave us a breakdown of the number of CAM adverts that they have been alerted to for breaking the British Code of Advertising in the last three years. These are shown in Table 4.

Table 4: Complaints Against Advertisements

	1998	**1999**	**2000***
Total number of complaints received by the ASA	12,052	12,141	8,542
Number of complaints received about 'alternative therapies'	153	157	84
Number of advertisements these complaints referred to	129	148	76
Dealt-with informally (minor or technical Code breaches)	19	24	6
Formally investigated (with published adjudication)	24	36	11
Complaints recorded but not acted upon	110	97	67

* = 1 January – 30 September 2000.

8.55 They told us that "when unacceptable references to serious medical conditions appear in advertisements for alternative therapies, it is generally due to ignorance on the part of the therapist about what is, and is not, acceptable within advertising. If an advertisement is published in a newspaper or magazine it is the responsibility of the publisher to check that it complies with the Code's rules. In most cases, acceptable advertising copy will be agreed before the advertisement is printed. Problematical claims within this sector tend to appear in leaflets and brochures that are written and produced by therapists themselves. These are much more difficult for the ASA, or other authority, to regulate" (p 390).

8.56 The ASA also told us: "Evidence provided to the Committee by the Consumers' Association (CA) stated that: "In terms of advertising in health generally...we have some concerns about the appropriateness of using advertising as a means of conveying information". This indicates a profound misunderstanding of the role and nature of advertising which largely constitutes brand advocacy and, by its very nature, is partial. Advertising is purchased specifically to present advertisers' views about their product, service or brand. On the basis of our research and experience, it is clear that rational consumers in today's 'consumer society' recognise this. Advertising must be 'legal, decent, honest and truthful', it must not mislead, but it does not provide balanced, objective or full information" (p 389).

8.57 False claims in CAM advertisements and leaflets are a serious issue; but legislation exists to control such problems **We recommend that CAM regulatory bodies, whether statutory or voluntary, should remind their members of these laws and take disciplinary action against anyone who breaks them. Information leaflets produced by such bodies should provide evidence-based information about a therapy aimed at informing patients, and should not be aimed at selling therapies to patients.**

An Overarching Information Body?

8.58 One way of making sure that the public and the medical professions do have access to impartial, high-quality information is to have a national information source covering all of CAM. This is one role that NCCAM subsumes in the USA. Dr Stephen Straus told us: "A disproportionately large investment, approximately nine per cent of our funding at this point, is invested in this area. We have a newsletter. Most importantly, we have a web site which gets approximately 490,000 hits per month and we fund a special modification of the National Library of Medicine Medline database articulated in terms of complementary and alternative medicine which has approximately 180,000 reference articles already in it and we are meeting to enhance and expand that" (Q 1760). The reason behind NCCAM's high level of investment in providing information is that "The American public gets its information very much like the public in the United Kingdom...Part of the pressure to create our Center has been the need as well as the desire of the American public for more competent guidance as to what works and what is safe and what does not work and is not safe. We are developing fact-sheets around various therapies, we are doing evidence-based reviews, we are funding evidence-based reviews" (Q 1760).

8.59 He went on to explain that the aim of their service is to provide an objective information source. They do not see a role for themselves in commenting upon bad quality material or trying to challenge people who make false claims. Their attitude towards countering the misleading material that is published on various other web sites is that it is best to fund "research whose results will set the record straight" (Q 1762).

8.60 The Natural Medicines Society (NMS), a voluntary CAM consumer information body, told us that they thought there was a great need for a national CAM information resource: "Even more than in the United States we probably do need such a body. The United States, to some extent, or parts of the United States, are behind Europe on the whole in the availability of CAM therapies. We have a proliferation of them and we have a very large percentage of the population making some use…there is certainly so much activity and so much misunderstanding that a central body might very well be the focus that seems to be needed" (Q 1567).

8.61 The NMS felt that, in the United Kingdom, "It would be desirable, for example, to see a national helpline where patients and possibly their physicians could receive first-line information. This is a function that the Natural Medicines Society has been carrying out semi-formally for 10 or more years, but lack of funding makes it impossible to develop our service to the scale necessary to match public demand" (P 157).

8.62 We asked the NMS whether all CAM groups would co-operate in setting up and running such an office. They told us: "It may have to be done for them perhaps. They are not the most co-operative of people. There are those who I think would find it straightforward and would work with that because they have already done it, who would see the sense of combining efforts. If there are enough of those they can provide the information. If others want to go outside of that then in reality the press in the long run will be less likely to have recourse to them" (Q 1573).

8.63 Both the Department of Health and the BMA have called for practitioners of CAM to set the standard and provide reliable information sources for the public. We agree that the necessary expertise lies with the professional specialist. There are, however, two significant problems with this prescription.

8.64 Firstly, much of the evidence we have received has reinforced the view that CAM therapies are rarely co-ordinated unless, like osteopathy and chiropractic, they have become statutorily registered. Leaving the provision of information to fragmented groups would possibly extend the current confusion that has already been visited upon the public. It is difficult to see how unity of view could be maintained in an information resource when it is lacking on issues such as educational standards and philosophical differences. When the frequent resort to self-promotion among the fringe elements of CAM is added, then we are not confident that unregulated professions are now able to meet this challenge in the public interest, no matter how much they would like to. Secondly, a consistent theme in this report is the lack of research evidence and activity in CAM, and the poor academic infrastructure available to subject the tenets of the various CAM therapies to scrutiny. We consider it would be desirable to link the provision of information to the public with at least the beginnings of a process of enquiry about the basis of these therapies, with overt efforts at quality assessments and audit, with acknowledgements of the importance of public accountability, and above all with clear-thinking guidelines for the practice of each therapy. Such information would not be easy to compile and update without partnerships with other resources and facilities, notably academic, regulatory and professional.

8.65 Several witnesses (e.g. NHS Alliance Q 148) suggested that FIM was an ideal body to explore initiatives in this area. FIM told us that they are very keen that there is a major initiative in this area. "This certainly is an area we believe that we can work in and assist the process" (Q 83). However, for such an initiative to be successful they believe that there is a need for "a significant investment in that by Government centrally" (Q 83). They went on to say: "I do not think it is a satisfactory position that there is no central initiative on this area. We would be very keen to work with other partners — the Government and CAM bodies — to actually begin to address this deficiency. There is an awful lot of information out there but the quality of it is hugely variable" (Q 83).

8.66 RCCM also supported the case for a national body; but they were more cautious, pointing out that "It is a very major task. Just to give you a quick example, CISCOM adds about 500 papers a month, and that is increasing month on month. That is just published research. If you are going to talk about different therapies and their regulatory bodies and everything else, that is a very, very major task and one, I think, that the Americans have found extremely difficult too"(Q 152).

8.67 However, other bodies we heard from were less enthusiastic about funding an information body particularly dedicated to CAM. The BMA told us: "We feel that it is really up to the practitioners of CAM to devise their own bodies for this. Having said that, they should also feel free to draw upon the good and bad experiences that there have been within medicine and the other paramedical fields who have been involved in regulation and in provision of information for many years. There are models within organisations such as the General Medical Council and indeed the Medical Royal

Colleges which may be of help, including some elements of things best to avoid" (Q 355). "Clearly again in this it is a matter of developing mutual trust between what have in the past historically, sadly, been seen as two opponents, and genuinely trying to help one another to form a body which works and which you can each have confidence in" (Q 355).

8.68 The Department of Health were not supportive of the idea of a Government-funded central CAM information resource, although they did tell us that "Stressing the importance of information and making sure that consumers are clear about what is being provided to them and the choice of treatments available is the principle which underscores a lot of the Government's initiatives within the NHS. They want to see CAM follow that example" (Q 58). They firmly held the belief that this was the role of the practitioner and therapy organisations themselves and not a role for Government.

8.69 Yvette Cooper MP, Parliamentary Under Secretary of State for Public Health, explained to us that one of the Government's concerns about providing information on CAM is that in some areas "the information simply does not exist...there is a lack of evidence base" (Q 1886). She explained that this was a worry because if the Government provide information on CAMs the public may believe they are advocating the use of those therapies, and this is not what they want to be doing for therapies which do not have an adequate evidence base to back up their claims. She continued: "The NHS Kite Mark...is something the public would take as authoritative, in a way they might not if they were simply surfing the Internet or finding out information for themselves" (Q 1888). Yvette Cooper also stated that the Government feel that the lack of effective regulatory structures backing up some CAM therapies means the Department would have worries about being seen to promote those therapies: "I think it is an area where the result of the lack of appropriate regulation also provides a constraint...in terms of what we are able to inform people about" (Q 1888).

8.70 Despite these reservations, we support the idea of a centralised information body because the level of public interest in CAM is high, yet there is a large amount of confusing information in the public domain, almost all produced either by the press to provide a story, or by CAM practitioners themselves who naturally want to advertise their particular therapy. Therefore a neutral national information body could play a valuable role in protecting the public by giving them the information they need to make sensible, informed decisions. While we do not make formal recommendations on this issue, we believe it is one which deserves serious consideration.

8.71 For many people who are well-informed, or have already decided to accept a CAM treatment, the simple provision of information, such as the contact details of local practitioners, may be sufficient to satisfy their requirements. For the general public or medical staff who are curious about CAM, perhaps with interest stimulated by press coverage, recommendations from their friends, or inquiries from their patients, there is a gap in the information that is available from the NHS, their natural point of reference.

8.72 During our Inquiry we have become convinced of the growing public interest in CAM, and we feel that the Department of Health and the NHS should take a lead in guiding people (and doctors) through the vast array of variable quality information on CAM. The current position of the Department of Health appears to be one of devolving the responsibility to the representative bodies of CAM therapies, whose views may not be seen to be entirely impartial, or the public media, whose coverage of CAM is often criticised, or to individual GPs or PCGs, each of whom scarcely has the time to find out about all of the various branches of CAM available. There is a need, in the words of Dr Straus, for more competent guidance as to what works and what is safe and what does not work and what is not safe (see para 8.58). Only then will the other types of information, such as points of contact, places to look for the results of further research, and lists of what various qualifications mean, be of value.

8.73 The natural place for people in the United Kingdom to turn to for health advice is the NHS, and we feel it is not adequately fulfilling its responsibilities in this area with regard to CAM. However, we are encouraged by the developments of the electronic National Health Library and NHS Direct, both of which seem ideally placed to fill the gaps in the NHS's CAM information provision as part of their wider remits. We urge that they do so speedily, and seek the advice of FIM which is well-placed to assist.

CHAPTER 9: DELIVERY

Current Patterns of Delivery

9.1 The majority of CAM is practised in the private sector. It is often accessed without referral from a GP, by patients who have read about treatments or have been told by friends of a certain practitioner, and who contact that practitioner directly and pay out of their own pocket. FIM confirmed that this was a common method of accessing CAM. They told us that "...a significant amount of complementary therapy is bought privately by people who can afford to buy it"(Q 109).

9.2 However CAM is also available on the NHS, and has been since its inception. The Department of Health commissioned an independent study in 1995 to help develop a picture of CAM access via general practice[53]. This study reported that 40% of GP partnerships in England provide access to CAM for NHS patients. But evidence shows that this provision is very patchy - whether patients have NHS access to CAM is dependent on the attitude of their particular PCG or Primary Care Trust (PCT)[54] (Q 109). FIM told us: "The Foundation's integrated health awards identified 80 good examples of integration both with primary and hospital services. It demonstrated that provision is increasingly becoming available through the NHS but access to such services is patchy" (P 30).

9.3 The NHS Confederation echoed these sentiments: They told that they support moves towards integration and that "This is a process that is already happening and the boundaries of what is considered "conventional" and "complementary" are constantly shifting (acupuncture in pain clinics, for example). Much of its foothold is, however, tenuous"(P 145).

9.4 The reaction of many of our witnesses to the patchiness of CAM provision on the NHS mirrors that which has been stimulated in the general public by "post-code prescribing". FIM told us "...if it is available for some people in the NHS, it should be available for all people through the NHS" (Q 111).

Methods of Delivery

9.5 Provision of CAM outside the NHS can be offered through many different mechanisms, including: access through health clubs and beauty parlours, over-the-counter self-medication; directly approaching and paying an independent CAM practitioner; self-referral to a specialist centre; and obtaining a GP referral to an independent CAM practitioner or specialist centre, whether paid for directly or through health insurance.

9.6 Unlike private CAM delivery, all NHS CAM has to be accessed through a GP or another member of the primary healthcare team. These methods for NHS referrals are outlined in Box 12. Currently most NHS CAM is delivered within primary care, although in some cases CAM is now part of secondary care (see paras 9.15-9.20)

9.7 The Department of Health's evidence to us was keen to emphasise that CAM practitioners are also welcome to try to play a role in supporting community health initiatives such as their Healthy Workplace Initiative, the Healthy Living Centres and Healthy Schools projects.

---

[53]   Thomas et al (1995) *National Survey of Access to Complementary Health via General Practice* University of Sheffield.

[54]   A PCT differs from a PCG in that it is legally responsible for the delivery of primary care services, unlike a PCG which is a sub-committee of a Health Authority. Most PCGs expect to develop into PCTs over the next 5 years.

Box 12

Methods of Delivery Within the NHS

PATIENT

GENERAL PRACTITIONER (or other member of primary care team)

may provide CAM treatment themselves if trained; or

↓ refer to

(a) A member of an on-site multi-disciplinary team (as in the Marylebone Health Centre)

(b) A specialist CAM centre within an NHS Acute Trust (e.g. London Homeopathic Hospital)

(c) A specialist CAM centre contracted by the District Health Authority (e.g. Centre for Complementary Health Studies in Southampton)

(d) An individual, off-site, CAM practitioner contracted by the Primary Care Group or Primary Care Trust

(e) A secondary care service within the NHS Acute Trust that uses CAM (as in some physiotherapy and orthopaedic clinics)

(f) If patient is terminally ill refer to a palliative care unit which provides CAM

(g) Take advantage of District Health Authority Initiatives that may be piloting CAM projects.

NB: A secondary or tertiary care specialist could also make these referrals.

Integrated Healthcare

9.8 When designing an integrated healthcare service, there are some basic questions that need to be considered. We visited the Marylebone Health Centre, an inner-city NHS GP practice with a multi-disciplinary team including CAM practitioners (see Appendix 4). There, Dr David Peters described the six stages of integrating CAM into general practice and discussed the main questions to be tackled at each stage. These were:

(i) Practice review – Which needs are being poorly met?

(ii) Resource assessment – Is CAM relevant? What is its evidence base? Is integration feasible?

(iii) Designing a service – Asking how will GPs use the service? What will be its aims? How will complementary practitioners be integrated into the primary care team?

(iv) Delivering the service – Developing referral procedures and working on resource monitoring.

(v) Management servicing – Including quality assurance procedures and evaluating outcomes,

(vi) Modifying the service in response to experience.

(vii) Once modification has taken place the steps can start all over again so the service is constantly self-monitoring and improving.

9.9 In terms of step 3 of this model, designing a service, this is a very important issue for all NHS integrative healthcare; no matter which delivery model is used it is very important to decide when GPs should consider a CAM referral. At the Marylebone Health Centre it was decided that GPs would refer to a CAM practitioner only for conditions where some evidence for the efficacy of a particular CAM existed. It was also decided that referrals would only take place if GPs wanted to refer, and if complementary practitioners thought they could help.

9.10 The Marylebone Health Centre developed a list of conditions that they commonly consider for CAM referrals. These include complex chronic illnesses such as: chronic fatigue syndrome; stress-related conditions; asthma; irritable bowel syndrome; eczema and non-specific allergies; back pain and migraine. GPs at the Centre consider a referral if there is an initial diagnosis of one of these conditions and if one of the following criteria applies: (a) conventional medicine has failed; (b) the patient is suffering side-effects from the conventional treatment; (c) the patient requests CAM for one of the conditions above; or (d) if the GP feels it is a complex case where a CAM may help (and having asked the CAM therapist they, too, feel they may be able to help.)

9.11 The other CAM practice we visited, the Southampton Centre for the Study of Complementary Medicine (see Appendix 5) was a very different organisation from the Marylebone Health Centre as it is an independent-provider organisation contracted by District Health Authorities to offer CAM services for specified conditions. However, the conditions for which it receives NHS referrals are very similar to those treated at the Marylebone Health Centre.

9.12 During our visit to Southampton they told us about a survey of the Centre which was published in the *British Medical Journal* which shows that most patients come with very long-term problems (average duration 10 years). The staff continuously audit their practice, and results for 1999 show impressive results for many patients suffering from chronic conditions, especially irritable bowel syndrome and myalgic encephalitis (ME), more often called the chronic fatigue syndrome.

9.13 The Southampton Centre for the Study of Complementary Medicine operates a contract with Dorset Area Health Authority. This is a unique arrangement within the NHS for CAM services and it operates in two parts. The first part is an integrated medicine unit which the Centre operates for one day each month at a GP practice in Dorset. GPs in local clinics are able to refer patients with any of six specific conditions to this clinic. These conditions are: chronic fatigue syndrome, irritable bowel syndrome, migraine, child behavioural problems, eczema and non-specific allergy. The second part of the contract with the Dorset Area Health Authority allows patients to travel to the Centre in Southampton for their treatment. Last year this resulted in 600 consultations. This system provides for the same six conditions as the first contract, although there is some flexibility. This service has proved to be quite popular with GPs, especially as a way of dealing with patients who are 'difficult' and whom they have been unable to help. The second part of the contract has been designed so that it is very easy to administer: it provides for six appointments for the specified condition, with the only formalities required being a letter of referral and a letter of progress to be sent to the referring GP. The six appointments can be extended if the GP writes to the Health Authority for permission. The Centre makes a conscious effort to make sure that GPs are always kept up-to-date about their patients' progress and treatment. This arrangement has allowed interested GPs to become fully informed about the methods that the Centre employs.

9.14 Both the Marylebone Health Centre and the Centre for the Study of Complementary Medicine are examples of integrative healthcare projects that GPs feel have benefited their patients and themselves. These provide evidence that there is a place for CAM in primary care, especially in the treatment of chronic conditions with which GPs often struggle to help their patients.

PRIMARY AND SECONDARY CARE

9.15 One of the questions that we have considered is whether CAM is more suited to primary or secondary healthcare delivery. Dr Michael Dixon of the NHS Alliance told us that in the delivery of CAM "...there is clearly a bias towards primary care... t is firmly in the primary care agenda already. I think also psychologically there is an empathy there, that is to say, first of all, both general practice, primary care and complementary medicine are holistic from their point of view, they are taking the whole person not just the constituent bits. Secondly, they are both very committed to the whole idea of self-care which secondary care often is not, it is often more the passive act of modern, traditional medicine. Thirdly, I think this whole concept of a therapeutic relationship is much stronger in primary than secondary care. There is a natural empathy in primary care" (Q 1474).

9.16 However, Professor Ruth Chambers, also from the NHS Alliance, added: "Without doubt we think it should also be in secondary care. We think it should be offered along all care pathways... so that the care pathway for back pain or whatever would automatically have complementary medicine featuring in the flow of a patient. It would be self-care: coming to the GP, going to secondary care and back again involving all the therapies. We think it should be a cost-effective option for reducing in-patient costs and that is why secondary care would be interested in learning more about it and adopting it where it fits" (Q 1474).

9.17 There are existing models of CAM being part of secondary care delivery, but they are limited to three or four main areas. First, where the manipulative therapies (osteopathy and chiropractic) have been integrated into orthopaedic care. Second, where acupuncture (and occasionally some of the relaxant therapies in Group 2) have been integrated into pain clinics. Third, where acupuncture and occasionally aromatherapy have been integrated into some obstetric and cancer services, and into palliative care, rehabilitation and care of the elderly. And fourth, where homeopathy is provided within secondary care through the homeopathic hospitals (see Appendix 6).

9.18 There are many different means through which CAM may be available on the NHS; definitive judgements cannot easily be made about which models are best as so little work has been done on evaluating this area. FIM told us that "...it is crucial that where there is successful integration of orthodox and CAM therapies that these projects are carefully evaluated" (p 30). This would help produce guidelines for future attempts at integration on issues such as when to refer, how to communicate about treatment regimes etc. FIM have recently received a small grant from the Department of Health to undertake some work in this area (p 30).

9.19 In conclusion, it seems that there are already several successful models of integration, although current levels of provision are patchy. In addition, with the recent introduction of Primary Care Groups and Trusts primary care delivery patterns are changing (this will be discussed in the next section). It is probably not necessary to ask which method of integrated healthcare is best but instead to ask which method of delivery is most appropriate in which situation? Work needs to be done to evaluate existing models of integration so that each new project can learn from those that came before. The anecdotal experiences brought to our attention seem to suggest that there is a valuable role for CAM in primary care, especially when provision concentrates on referrals for those conditions for which, according to our evidence, CAM helps most (e.g. chronic complaints, allergies).

9.20 **We recommend that those practising privately accessed CAM therapies should work towards integration between CAM and conventional medicine, and CAM therapists should encourage patients with conditions that have not been previously discussed with a medical practitioner to see their GP. We also urge CAM practitioners and GPs to keep an open mind about each other's ability to help their patients, to make patients feel comfortable about integrating their healthcare provision and to exchange information about treatment programmes and their perceptions of the healthcare needs of patients.**

Primary Care Groups

9.21 Prior to the introduction of PCGs in April 1999, GP fund-holding practices could support the provision of CAM services through savings they had achieved on their budgets, and an estimated 12% of fund-holding practices were choosing to do this in 1995[55]. Once PCGs were introduced, all practice-based services, including CAM services, came under review. Many of our witnesses expressed concern that fund-holding practices which had decided to 'go it alone' in providing CAM services would not be able to convince their new partners in a PCG that CAM provision should continue.

9.22 The Department of Health commissioned a study in April 2000 on the way CAM services are "reconfigured in the NHS under PCGs"[56]. This study identified the need for a consensus across the PCG as one important factor likely to determine CAM provision (previous evidence shows that consensus on CAM was hard to reach even when it was only sought within the individual practices). The study also explained that any decision about CAM will have to take into account the two guiding principles for PCGs: these are the need to take into account the issue of adequate clinical governance, and to concentrate on the local population's primary care needs.

9.23 There does seem to be some justification for CAM practitioners' concern that the organisation of PCGs will impair the prospects of CAM services being commissioned within the NHS. We took evidence from the NHS Alliance, which was formed as a result of the introduction of PCGs in order to represent them and help them to become established (Q 1459). They told us that the extent of commissioning of CAM did seem to be falling, and with particular reference to osteopathy (one of the CAM services most commonly commissioned under fund-holding) they told us that "...surveys suggest that PCGs are not renewing the existing contracts held over from former fundholding arrangements. Our own research indicates that over 32.8 per cent have been discontinued. We believe this is due to the fact that PCGs have been given the role of balancing inequality of access from the old fund-holding system. This means they have to make a decision as to whether to extend a minority service or discontinue it completely. The problem we face, and it is a very important one, is that by discontinuing osteopathy PCGs are reversing the trend for innovation within primary care" (Q 427).

---

[55] Thomas, K. & Luff, D. (April 2000) The Provision of Complementary Medicine Under Primary Care Groups: Interim Report to the Department of Health. Medical Care Research Unit, University of Sheffield.

[56] Thomas, K. & Luff, D. (2000) *(Op.cit.)*.

9.24 The NHS Alliance went on to elaborate on the problems CAM will face if PCGs continue with this trend: "If new approaches to treatment cannot be piloted in one or two GP practices before they are extended to all in a PCG then important opportunities for research in evidence-based practice will be lost. This reversal of the trend to using osteopathy in primary care will continue unless there is some incentive against it. Once this relationship is lost it is difficult to see how comparative studies will ever occur" (Q 427). They also suggested that one way of attempting to encourage PCGs to reverse this trend would be "…some exemption given to PCGs to allow the piloting of CAM projects within a single or a couple of GP units within each PCG. This would enable the evidence to be built up as to whether or not it is applicable to extend that service over the rest of the PCG. What we fear is that if that flexibility is not built into the system then complementary medicine will suffer" (Q 429).

9.25 The NHS Alliance did indicate that some of the problems discussed above may not be permanent: "… primary care groups and trusts are getting on to their feet. The primary care group is meant to be instilling new ideas, it is meant to be thinking the unthinkable, it is meant to be taking risks in many ways. There have not been great risks taken in that first year, largely, as I say, because of lack of funds. They will start, I think, taking greater risks in the conventional sense, I do not mean real risks of course. They will start doing that as they gain their confidence and their feet…as the public become more involved in what they are doing…It will take time for the professionals to become involved, it is going to take time for the patients to become involved, even more time for them to get properly briefed and be able to arm themselves with the same sorts of arguments and evidence that the professionals may be using against them. It is very doctor dominated at the moment, the scene, but I think that will change" (Q 1468).

9.26 However, some of the GPs interviewed in the Department of Health's commissioned report on the provision of complementary medicine under PCGs, referred to in paragraph 9.21, were less sure that the situation would change in the near future. That survey found that "most of the service providers who rated complementary medicine as a low priority within their PCG at the moment, felt that this situation was likely to continue in the medium to long term"[57].

9.27 The NHS Alliance told us that they did have a positive vision of how CAM may be provided by PCGs and PCTs in the future. Dr Michael Dixon told us: "I would see the future provision of complementary care being something that is decided at PCT level so that there is some standardisation and equity and that the actual service could be provided either from one of these centres or, where you have got large practices, there is no reason why the individual therapist should not be working in those practices. I think what that would offer would be a co-ordinated programme of complementary care within the Primary Care Trust and one which was flexible as to where the care was going to be provided…The new Primary Care Groups and Trusts are going to have to commission care, the long pathways of care, using these long-term service agreements. What I foresee is that the pathways of care, the long-term service agreements, will give relatively precise indications of at what point a patient might be offered a complementary option and, therefore, clear guidelines to all the primary care practitioners in that group as to when the work might be feasible or could be offered within the budget of that Primary Care Group. Therefore, again you would have that level of standardisation, whether the treatment was being offered from the resource centre centrally or whether it was being offered in an individual practice" (Q 1463).

9.28 The NHS Executive was commissioned by the Department of Health to produce a report on the key issues relating to CAM in Primary Care. The report was prepared by drawing together an information base on CAM in primary care through examining entries to the Guild of Health Writers' Integrated Healthcare Awards Competition, and through a questionnaire which was sent to all PCGs (and received a 60% response rate). The report identified some patterns of PCGs' commissioning of CAM therapies and important issues for PCGs to keep in mind. These were:

- CAM occupied a greater or lesser profile within the PCG depending on local circumstances, e.g. the financial state of the PCG, need to review continuation of existing services and having to balance PCG priorities

- Provision of CAM is usually based on the interest and enthusiasm of particular individuals rather than being part of an overall strategy of provision of services.

- Where no such therapies were being provided, about one-fifth of PCGs had plans for provision within the next 2-3 years.

- Factors to be taken into account in the provision of CAM were:

  a) information on effectiveness and cost effectiveness;

---

57 Thomas, K. & Luff, D (2000) (Op.cit.).

b) knowledge of accreditation procedures and standards for practitioners;

c) the wider resource implications of any decisions made.

- Patients do not necessarily see the NHS as their provider of access to CAM, but do see NHS healthcare professionals as an information resource.

- Given the significant number of people requesting and using CAM treatment it seems that doctors and healthcare professionals will not only need to be aware of what is available but also be able to give advice on existing evidence.

9.29 Within this research work[58] several areas for further work to aid PCGs in making informed decisions about CAM were identified. In response to these needs the Department of Health, the NHS Executive and the National Association of Primary Care collaborated to put together and publish a *Complementary Medicine Information Pack for Primary Care Groups* in June 2000. The aim of this pack is to "give primary care groups a basic reference on complementary and alternative therapies most commonly provided by PCGs." It includes information on current levels of provision, on individual therapies and the groups representing them on how to make referrals to CAM practitioners, and it outlines existing models of provision as well as identifying further sources of information. As these were all areas identified by PCGs as issues upon which they needed guidance it will, we hope, be a useful resource for PCGs in their practice reviews.

9.30 Another factor that is likely to impact on PCGs' commissioning patterns is the local Health Improvement Programme. The Department of Health told us that "Health Improvement Programmes (HImP) will be the local strategy for improving health and healthcare. They will cover the most important health needs of the local population, and how these are to be met by the NHS and its partner organisations...HImPs that engage all local interests and which will result in comprehensive LTSAs [Long-Term Service Arrangements - the replacement of annual contracts as the means of commissioning services] will take time to develop fully. As LTSAs develop, patients and their representative groups will be able to take an active role in influencing commissioning decisions. Those responsible for commissioning healthcare services will be required to involve users and carers in identifying local priorities...If local people and the relevant Primary Care Group, Health Authority and NHS Trust feel strongly that there is a priority need for CAM services, those responsible for commissioning services will need to consider whether these would represent a cost-effective means of meeting local health needs, consistent with the objectives of the local HImP" (P 117).

9.31 The newly published *Complementary Medicine Information Pack for Primary Care Groups*[59], previously mentioned, also discusses the role of HImPs in determining the use of CAM by PCGs. It advises that "Whilst CAM may not be specifically mentioned in the PCG Health Improvement Plan or Primary Care Investment Plan (PCIP), the PCG could still have an interest in how CAM may be integrated into services to improve the health of the local population. Across the PCG, there will probably be some variation in the extent to which the local population may be able to access CAM, usually related more to differences in local provision rather than patient need. In these circumstances the PCG will want to consider how the issue of equity of access for the local population should be addressed...A commissioning model for PCGs could involve care pathways for a given condition rather than individual services, providing an opportunity for CAM to be used and incorporated as an option, especially where there is evidence of efficacy to support its use."

Gatekeeper Role of GPs

9.32 The gatekeeper role of GPs is traditionally the route to most specialist care on the NHS; as Box 12 showed, all NHS CAM provision is currently accessed either through GP referral or the referral of another member of the primary or secondary healthcare team. As discussed earlier in this report, one of the main dangers of CAM is that patients could miss out on conventional medical diagnosis and treatment because they approached a CAM practitioner first who did not have the comprehensive medical training of a medical practitioner. One way of ensuring that this risk is minimised is to have GPs acting as gatekeepers so that CAM therapies can only be accessed (on the NHS) if the patient is referred by their GP or another member of the primary healthcare team.

9.33 The Royal College of General Practitioners (RCGP) supported the GP gatekeeper as the route for CAM access on the NHS. They told us: "The GP is the gatekeeper for many other services and, of course, if the patient has a particular condition, then in theory there is no reason why one should not consider CAM therapy as one of the points of referral...People also see the GP as somebody who can look at the effectiveness of what is likely to work for a particular condition. It may be a little bit

---

58 Thomas, K. & Luff, D. (2000) *(Op.cit.)*.
59 Thomas, K. & Luff, D. (2000) *(Op.cit.)*.

difficult to work out the full benefits of a particular treatment without having a full assessment. It may just be the initial assessment but in some way co-ordinated" (QQ 1484 & 1490).

9.34 The BMA also envisaged the gatekeeper role as the best route for CAM access on the NHS: "We would anticipate that gatekeeper role within the NHS function. So if we are going to refer or delegate at the expense of the NHS we would expect it to be the route into that" (Q 378).

9.35 The gatekeeper role of the GP or other member of the primary healthcare team not only minimises the risk of failing to diagnose serious problems but also ensures that the GP is aware of the treatment their patient is getting, and that all treatment is recorded in patient records. It also encourages communication between healthcare professionals. Dr Simon Fradd of the BMA also saw advantages in the gatekeeper role for financial reasons: "The reason, I would say, for that gatekeeper role within the NHS is because we have finite resources and we have to balance that. This comes back to the whole evidence base again. In my own commissioning group in Nottingham we had to make a decision: would we buy CAM procedures or would we buy more hip replacements? In the lack of really clear evidence we bought the hip replacements. I have a function, not just in clinical gatekeeping but in financial gatekeeping, and that is why I see a need for a gatekeeper role within the NHS" (Q 379).

9.36 The gatekeeper role can only be effective in relation to NHS CAM provision. In the private sector it would be virtually impossible to have such a requirement to control CAM access. Even if it were possible, it is unlikely that it would be desirable. If people wish to access CAM practitioners without a GP referral, this is their right, as long as they are doing so privately. In fact, such visits probably aid the NHS, reducing the burden on an already over-burdened service. If all such patients were required to go through their GP it would add more pressure upon busy doctors. However, this does mean that if patients access CAM privately they may either: (i) not approach a GP first when they could be seriously ill and may benefit from conventional treatment; or (ii) they may see their GP but not tell him/her they are also having CAM treatment, which may interfere with the treatment which the doctors provide. Therefore it is very important that CAM practitioners encourage their patients to see their GP about health problems for which they have not sought a medical opinion beforehand. It is also important that GPs do not make patients feel embarrassed about accessing CAM treatments, but instead encourage openness so as to work with the CAM practitioner communicating about the patient's progress, etc. The BMA agreed with this approach, saying they would encourage "…best practice so that there is communication from the CAM practitioner to the patient's family doctor, and that would be the very least. However, I do not think we need to be proscriptive about it, but we do need the quality controls that we have spent quite a lot of time talking about today, to protect the public. Also, we need to make it clear to the public that the medical profession are behind this; that the public need not feel embarrassed about using an alternative practitioner" (Q 378).

9.37 **We recommend that all NHS provision of CAM should continue to be through GP referral (or by referral from doctors or other healthcare professionals working in primary, secondary or tertiary care).**

Criteria for NHS Provision

9.38 One of the questions in our Call for Evidence asked what level of evidence was needed to justify NHS provision of CAM.

9.39 We heard much evidence about this matter. Many submissions suggested that 'only CAM therapies with an adequate evidence base in their favour should be considered for NHS integration.' As we discussed in Chapter 3, this is a difficult principle to apply as an adequate evidence base is hard to define. The Royal London Homoeopathic Hospital recognised this was a problem and told us: "As a general rule only therapies which have some evidence in their support should be introduced, but this should be interpreted flexibly: it may be necessary to introduce a therapy with a weak evidence base in NHS settings before it can be adequately evaluated. Conversely, existing evidence may not be generalisable to NHS contexts. It would be difficult to define minimum required standards of evidence in a hard and fast manner" (P 195).

9.40 In the NHS Executive's study on key issues for CAM in Primary Care[60] discussed in the previous section, one of the questions put to the PCGs in the survey was: "What factors are important in decision-making on the provision of complementary therapies throughout the PCG?" Respondents were asked to identify the five most important factors, and the results show that in considering CAM's role in NHS primary care the most important factors are evidence of effectiveness and cost-effectiveness, followed by accreditation procedures and standards (See Figure 1).

---

[60]   Thomas, K. and Luff, D. (2000) *(Op.cit.)*.

Figure 1:

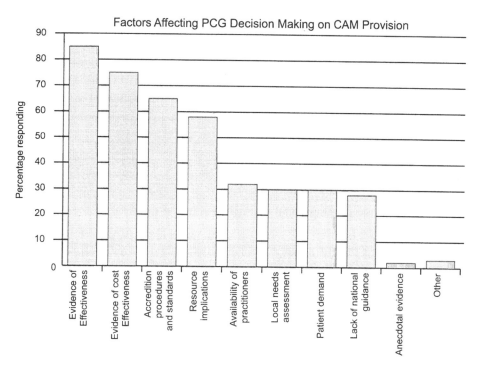

9.41 These findings again stress the importance of doing more research and gathering more evidence about CAM's effectiveness, as has been discussed in previous chapters. But the Royal London Homoeopathic Hospital's point that it may be necessary to introduce into the NHS new therapies with weak evidence bases in order to facilitate such research was reiterated by other witnesses.

9.42 The NHS Confederation told us "Integration in itself will also assist in the process of developing an evidence base. It is also the most promising way to take forward the matter of public provision. The NHS Confederation believes there are several service reasons why CAM should be publicly funded. However it should be made clear that in the current financial climate, provision of CAM in the NHS would have to compete with other priorities. It is likely that these services not backed by good evidence will be given a low priority" (P 145).

9.43 The NHS Confederation believes that there are several steps to be taken in deciding the extent of future provision of CAM. These are:

- "Systematically appraising the evidence and emerging evidence…alongside any other health technology assessments. NICE should take the lead in such appraisals.

- "Where an appraisal is promising yet sufficient evidence is not available…supporting further research and development work" (P 145).

9.44 One of the prime reasons for integrating CAM into the NHS will be if it is found to be cost-effective and can save scarce medical resources. We have heard some evidence that preliminary studies show that integrated healthcare can be cheaper than conventional medicine alone but more work needs to be done in this area. FIM told us: "The amount of work which is done on cost-effectiveness within the NHS is very limited, similarly, there is very little which has been done in terms of the cost-effectiveness of CAM provision. There are some findings to show that it did result in savings to the NHS. Our view would be that cost-effectiveness is an area of additional research which should be given attention, for example, across some of the chronic conditions which could be alleviated by CAM approaches. We would suggest that certainly more research needs to be done in this area. It is a very important one" (Q 112).

9.45 There are also questions of what level of regulation a therapy, or a practitioner, should be subject to if they are to work on the NHS. This was discussed in Chapter 5 on Regulation

9.46 **We recommend that only those CAM therapies which are statutorily regulated, or have a powerful mechanism of voluntary self-regulation, should be made available, by reference from doctors and other healthcare professionals working in primary, secondary or tertiary care, on the NHS.**

SUMMARY OF RECOMMENDATIONS

Many of our recommendations make reference to the way we have organised therapies into three separate groups in the Report. These groupings are outlined in detail in Chapter 2 but for ease of reference a short synopsis of our grouping system is as follows:

- *The first group* embraces what may be called the principal disciplines, two of which, osteopathy and chiropractic, are already regulated in their professional activity and education by Acts of Parliament. The others are acupuncture, herbal medicine and homeopathy. Each of these therapies claims to have an individual diagnostic approach and are seen as the 'Big 5' by most of the CAM world.

- *The second group* contains therapies which are most often used to complement conventional medicine and do not purport to embrace diagnostic skills. It includes aromatherapy; the Alexander Technique; body work therapies, including massage; counselling, stress therapy; hypnotherapy; reflexology and probably shiatsu, meditation and healing.

- *The third group* embraces those other disciplines which purport to offer diagnostic information as well as treatment and which, in general, favour a philosophical approach and are indifferent to the scientific principles of conventional medicine, and through which various and disparate frameworks of disease causation and its management are proposed. These therapies can be split into two sub-groups: Group 3a includes long-established and traditional systems of healthcare such as Ayurvedic medicine and Traditional Chinese medicine. Group 3b covers other alternative disciplines which lack any credible evidence base such as crystal therapy, iridology, radionics, dowsing and kinesiology.

Introduction (Chapter 1)

1. More detailed quantitative information is required on the levels of CAM use in the United Kingdom, in order to inform the public and healthcare policy-makers, and we recommend that suitable national studies be commissioned to obtain this information (para 1.21).

Evidence (Chapter 4)

2. Diagnostic procedures must be reliable and reproducible and more attention must be paid to whether CAM diagnostic procedures, as well as CAM therapies, have been scientifically validated. We agree that this is an issue that should always be kept in mind when doing research in this area (para 4.16).

3. In our opinion any therapy that makes specific claims for being able to treat specific conditions should have evidence of being able to do this above and beyond the placebo effect. This is especially true for therapies which aim to be available on the NHS and aim to operate as an alternative to conventional medicine, specifically therapies in Group 1. The therapies in our Groups 3a and b also aim to operate as an alternative to conventional medicine, and have sparse, or non-existent, evidence bases. Those therapies in our Group 2 which aim to operate as an adjunct to conventional medicine, and mainly make claims in the area of relaxation and stress management, are in lesser need of proof of treatment-specific effects but should control their claims according to the evidence available to them (para 4.18).

4. We recommend that if a therapy does gain a critical mass of evidence to support its efficacy, then the NHS and the medical profession should ensure that the public have access to it and its potential benefits (para 4.37).

Regulation (Chapter 5)

5. We recommend that, in order to protect the public, professions with more than one regulatory body make a concerted effort to bring their various bodies together and to develop a clear professional structure (para 5.12).

6. We recommend that each of the therapies in Group 2 should organise themselves under a single professional body for each therapy. These bodies should be well promoted so that the public who access these therapies are aware of them. Each should comply with core professional principles, and relevant information about each body should be made known to medical practitioners and other healthcare professionals. Patients could then have a single, reliable point of reference for standards,

and would be protected against the risk of poorly-trained practitioners and have redress for poor service (para 5.23).

7. It is our opinion that acupuncture and herbal medicine are the two therapies which are at a stage where it would be of benefit to them and their patients if the practitioners strive for statutory regulation under the Health Act 1999, and we recommend that they should do so. Statutory regulation may also be appropriate eventually for the non-medical homeopaths. Other professions must strive to come together under one voluntary self-regulating body with the appropriate features outlined in Box 5, and some may wish ultimately to aim to move towards regulation under the Health Act once they are unified with a single voice (paras 5.53 and 5.55).

8. We recommend that each existing regulatory body in the healthcare professions should develop clear guidelines on competency and training for their members on the position they take in relation to their members' activities in well organised CAM disciplines; as well as guidelines on appropriate training courses and other relevant issues. In drawing up such guidelines the conventional regulatory bodies should communicate with the relevant complementary regulatory bodies and the Foundation for Integrated Medicine to obtain advice on training and best practice and to encourage integrated practice (para 5.79).

9. We encourage the bodies representing medical and non-medical CAM therapists, particularly those in our Groups 1 and 2, to collaborate more closely, especially on developing reliable public information sources. We recommend that if CAM is to be practised by any conventional healthcare practitioners, they should be trained to standards comparable to those set out for that particular therapy by the appropriate (single) CAM regulatory body (para 5.83).

10. We recommend that the MCA find a mechanism that would allow members of the public to identify health products that had met the stringent requirements of licensing and to differentiate them from unregulated competitors. This should be accompanied by strong enforcement of the law in regard to products that might additionally confuse the customer with claims and labelling that resemble those permitted by marketing authorisations (para 5.93).

11. We strongly recommend that the Government should maintain their effective advocacy of a new regulatory framework for herbal medicines in the United Kingdom and the rest of the European Union, and urge all parties to ensure that new regulations adequately reflect the complexities of the unregulated sector (para 5.95).

12. We are concerned about the safety implications of an unregulated herbal sector and we urge that all legislative avenues be explored to ensure better control of this unregulated sector in the interests of the public health (para 5.97).

13. We support the view that any new regulatory regime should respect the diversity of products used by herbal practitioners and allow for simplified registration of practitioner stocks. Nevertheless, any such regime must ensure that levels of quality and assurance of safety are not compromised (para 5.98).

Professional Training and Education (Chapter 6)

14. Establishing an independent accreditation board along the lines of the British Acupuncture Accreditation Board is a positive move. Other therapies with fragmented professional representation may wish to use this as a model (para 6.20).

15. We recommend that CAM training courses should become more standardised and be accredited and validated by the appropriate professional bodies. All those who deliver CAM treatments, whether conventional health professionals or CAM professionals, should have received training in that discipline independently accredited by the appropriate regulatory body (para 6.33).

16. We suggest that the CAM therapies, particularly those in our Groups 1 and 2, should identify Continuing Professional Development in practice as a core requirement for their members (para 6.34).

17. We consider that it is imperative that higher educational institutions and any regulatory bodies in CAM liaise in order to ensure that training is adequate for registration. If extra training is required after academic qualification to ensure fitness to practise, this should be defined by the appropriate professional body, which should then implement appropriate mechanisms in order to see that this objective is achieved (para 6.40).

18. We recommend that training in anatomy, physiology and basic biochemistry and pharmacology should be included within the education of practitioners of therapies that are likely to offer diagnostic information, such as the therapies in Groups 1 and 3a. Although it may be useful for other therapists to understand basic biomedical science, there is no requirement for such in-depth understanding if the therapy being practised is to be used as an adjunct to conventional medicine (para 6.43).

19. We recommend that every therapist working in CAM should have a clear understanding of the principles of evidence-based medicine and healthcare. This should be a part of the curriculum of all

CAM therapy courses. An in-depth understanding of research methods may be even more important for those therapies that operate independently of medical supervision, and which attempt to make a diagnosis and to cure complaints rather than for those which offer relaxation or aim to improve the general quality of life of patients. Therefore training in research and statistical methods may be particularly appropriate for practitioners of therapies in Groups 1 and 3a. But we consider that an understanding of research methods and outcomes should be included in the training of all CAM practitioners. It is important that all of those teaching these courses should understand these principles (para 6.49).

20. We recommend that all CAM training defines limits of the particular therapist's competence as clearly as possible in the state of current knowledge. Training should also give students clear guidance on when a patient should be referred to a primary care physician or even directly to secondary hospital care (para 6.52).

21. We recommend that all CAM therapists should be made aware of the other CAM therapies available to their patients and how they are practised. We do not think it should be assumed that CAM practitioners competent in one discipline necessarily understand the others (para 6.54).

22. We conclude that there should be flexibility for training institutions to decide how to educate practitioners. It is the relevant professional regulatory body of a specific CAM therapy that should set objectives of training and define core competencies appropriate to their particular discipline, and we so recommend. We do not advocate a blanket core curriculum (para 6.61).

23. We recommend that, whether subject to statutory or voluntary regulation, all healthcare regulatory bodies should consider the relevance to their respective professions of those elements set out in paragraph 6.55 (para 6.62).

24. We recommend that therapies with a fragmented professional organisation work with Healthwork UK to develop National Occupational Standards, and we encourage the Department of Health to further support Healthwork UK's activity with such therapies; we believe that this would be of long-term benefit to the public (para 6.70).

25. We recommend that familiarisation should prepare medical students for dealing with patients who are either accessing CAM or have an interest in doing so. This familiarisation should cover the potential uses of CAM, the procedures involved, their potential benefits and their main weaknesses and dangers (para 6.77).

26. We recommend that every medical school ensures that all their medical undergraduates are exposed to a level of CAM familiarisation that makes them aware of the choices their patients might make (para 6.79).

27. We recommend that Royal Colleges and other training authorities in the healthcare field should address the issue of familiarisation with CAM therapies among doctors, dentists and veterinary surgeons by supporting appropriate Continuing Professional Development opportunities (para 6.85).

28. The General Osteopathic and Chiropractic Councils, and any other regulatory bodies, should develop schemes whereby they accredit certain training courses aimed specifically at doctors and other healthcare professionals, and which are developed in conjunction with them. Similar schemes should be pursued by dentists and veterinary surgeons (para 6.95).

29. We recommend that the UKCC work with the Royal College of Nursing to make CAM familiarisation a part of the undergraduate nursing curriculum and a standard competency expected of qualified nurses, so that they are aware of the choices that their patients may make. We would also expect nurses specialising in areas where CAM is especially relevant (such as palliative care) to be made aware of any CAM issues particularly pertinent to that speciality during their postgraduate training. The Royal College of Nursing and the UKCC, as they do not provide CAM training themselves, should compile a list of courses in CAM that they approve, in order that nurses who wish to practise in this field can obtain guidance on appropriate training (para 6.106).

Research (Chapter 7)

30. To conduct research into the CAM disciplines will require much work and resources, and will therefore be time-consuming. Hence, we recommend that three questions should be prioritised and addressed in the following order:

- To provide a starting point for possible improvements in CAM treatment, to show whether further inquiry would be useful, and to highlight any areas where its application could inform conventional medicine does the treatment offer therapeutic benefits greater than placebo?

- To protect patients from hazardous practices – is the treatment safe?

- To help patients, doctors and healthcare administrators choose whether or not to adopt the treatment – how does it compare, in medical outcome and cost-effectiveness, with other forms of treatment? (para 7.7)

31. We recommend that CAM practitioners and researchers should attempt to build up an evidence base with the same rigour as is required of conventional medicine, using both RCTs and other research designs (para 7.26).

32. To achieve equity with more conventional proposals, we recommend that research funding agencies should build up a database of appropriately trained individuals who understand CAM practice. The research funding agencies could then use these individuals as members of selection panels and committees or as external referees as appropriate (para 7.45).

33. We recommend that universities and other higher education institutions provide the basis for a more robust research infrastructure in which CAM and conventional research and practice can take place side-by-side and can benefit from interaction and greater mutual understanding. We recommend that a small number of such centres of excellence, in or linked to medical schools, be established with the support of research funding agencies including the Research Councils, the Department of Health, Higher Education Funding Councils and the charitable sector (para 7.57).

34. Bodies such as the Departments of Health, the Research Councils and the Wellcome Trust should help to promote a research culture in CAM by ensuring that the CAM world is aware of the opportunities they offer. The Department of Health should exercise a co-ordinating role. Limited funds should be specifically aimed at training CAM practitioners in research methods. As many CAM practitioners work in the private sector and cannot afford to train in research, we recommend that a number of university-based academic posts, offering time for research and teaching, should be established (para 7.67).

35. We recommend that companies producing products used in CAM should invest more heavily in research and development (para 7.81).

36. We recommend that the NHS R&D directorate and the MRC should pump-prime this area with dedicated research funding in order to create a few centres of excellence for conducting CAM research, integrated with research into conventional healthcare. This will also help to promote research leadership and an evaluative research culture in CAM. Such funds should support research training fellowships and a limited number of high-quality research projects. This initiative should be sufficient to attract high-quality researchers and to enable them both to carry out large-scale studies and to continue to train CAM researchers in this area within a multi-disciplinary environment. We believe ten years would be sufficient for the pump-priming initiative as, for example, in the case of some MRC programme grants and various training and career development awards available in conventional medicine. The Association of Medical Research Charities may also like to follow this example (para 7.102).

Information (Chapter 8)

37. We recommend that the NHS Centre for Reviews and Dissemination work with the RCCM, the UK Cochrane Centre, and the British Library to develop a comprehensive information source with the help of the CISCOM database, in order to provide comprehensive and publicly available information sources on CAM research, and that resources be made available to enable these organisations to do so (para 8.21).

38. We see the NHS as the natural home in the United Kingdom for reliable, non-promotional information on all types of healthcare; providing such a home is particularly important for CAM, where the diversity of opinion and organisations make it almost impossible for individuals to gain an overview. Consequently we support the plans of the Department of Health to make information on CAM available through NHS Direct, and we urge that they be carried out in the very near future. We recommend that the information should contain not only contact details of the relevant bodies and a list of NHS provision of CAM in each local area, but also some guidance to help patients (and their doctors) evaluate different CAM therapies (para 8.31).

39. We are aware that the National electronic Health Library and NHS Direct Online plan to have information available about CAM in the future and we support these plans and recommend that they are carried forward (para 8.48).

40. We recommend that CAM regulatory bodies, whether statutory or voluntary, remind their members of the laws concerning false claims in advertisements and take disciplinary action against anyone who breaks them. Information leaflets produced by such bodies should provide evidence-based information about a therapy aimed at informing patients, and should not be aimed at selling therapies to patients (para 8.57).

Delivery (Chapter 9)

41. We recommend that those practising privately-accessed CAM therapies should work towards integration between CAM and conventional medicine, and CAM therapists should encourage patients with conditions that have not been previously discussed with a medical practitioner to see their GP. We also urge CAM practitioners and GPs to keep an open mind about each other's ability to help their patients, to make patients feel comfortable about integrating their healthcare provision and to exchange information about treatment programmes and their perceptions of the healthcare needs of patients (para 9.20).

42. We recommend that all NHS provision of CAM should continue to be through GP referral (or by referral from doctors or other healthcare professionals working in primary, secondary or tertiary care) (para 9.37).

43. We recommend that only those CAM therapies which are statutory regulated, or have a powerful mechanism of voluntary self-regulation, should be made available, by reference from doctors and other healthcare professionals working in primary, secondary or tertiary care, on the NHS (para 9.46).

APPENDIX 1

Difficulties of Randomised Controlled Trials (see para 7.25)

Concerns over RCTs distorting a therapy or disguising its efficacy are not the unique concerns of CAM practitioners. Vincent & Furnham suggest that as attempts to apply the RCT to a wider and wider range of treatments have occurred, more and more problems have been uncovered. They list 10 such problems:

(i) "Problems may arise because subjects randomised to different treatment groups may meet and discuss their treatment. Assignment to natural groups (e.g. comparison of two school districts) may be preferable to randomisation.

(ii) Blinding may not be feasible for some treatments...there is no clear equivalent to placebo drugs for some treatments.

(iii) Participation in a study may affect the behaviour of people taking part. Simply being monitored and assessed regularly may have a beneficial effect...

(iv) Subjects agreeing to take part in a trial may not be typical of the general population of patients with that particular problem. Entry criteria are strict to ensure comparability between groups...Patients with atypical symptoms, multiple problems or a poor prognosis may be excluded.

(v) Reduced compliance with treatment because of the possibility of receiving placebo treatment may arise.

(vi) Using standard treatments in the trial may sometimes be in a sense artificial and may have little relevance to clinical practice. Treatment within the context of a controlled trial may have to be precisely specified at the outset, which inhibits a more flexible patient-centred approach. The trial may therefore not be a true test of the therapy as used in clinical practice and the needs of the patient may conflict with the requirements of research.

(vii) Individual variations in response are often ignored in an analysis that only considers average group responses. Patients who are made worse by the treatment may not be given enough attention in reports...

(viii) Ethical problems may arise in a variety of contexts, particularly where placebo treatments are involved, or the patient or clinician has a marked preference for one treatment option over another. These concerns increase when the disease is potentially disabling or life-threatening.

(ix) The main outcome measure, based on clinical assessment and objective tests, may not reflect the patients' perspectives of what constitutes an important and beneficial change. Patients may be more concerned with the quality of their lives, which may not be closely linked with changes in biochemical parameters or other disease indicators. However, quality-of-life measures are now much more widely used.

(x) The concern with eliminating the placebo effect when assessing a treatment in relation to a comparable placebo may mean that important psychological variables are neglected."

All these methodological issues apply to both conventional and CAM treatment trials. Therefore CAM is not necessarily a special case requiring radically new methodologies.

APPENDIX 2

Features of the General Osteopathic Council and the General Chiropractic Council

The General Osteopathic Council

The GOsC was established under the Osteopaths Act 1993 to regulate, develop and promote the profession. It is the only body, by statute, able to register and regulate osteopathic practitioners by law. It is a criminal offence for anyone to practise as an "osteopath" unless they are registered with the General Osteopathic Council.

The GOsC has a duty to safeguard patients by ensuring high standards of ethical and clinical practice. Osteopathy was the first healthcare profession to be awarded statutory self-regulation for over 40 years, and the first of the professions previously outside conventional medical services to achieve statutory recognition.

The Act came fully into force in May 2000. It will ensure that:

All osteopaths have proven high standards of clinical competence.

High standards of professional conduct are enforced by a single regulatory body.

All osteopaths have professional indemnity insurance.

There is an effective mechanism for dealing with complaints.

The Act established four Statutory Committees:

The *Education Committee,* committed to training and maintaining the highest standards of osteopathic education and practice for the benefit of the public.

The *Investigating Committee*, which will investigate any allegations against a registered osteopath of conduct which falls short of the standards required.

The *Professional Conduct Committee,* which will consider allegations of professional misconduct referred to it by the Investigating Committee.

The *Health Committee,* which will consider allegations of serious impairment due to ill-health of a registered osteopath referred to it by the Investigating Committee.

In addition to these Statutory Committees there are a number of other committees covering executive matters such as legal issues and finance, ethics and external affairs.

The Statutory Register opened on 9 May 1998. Closure of the initial period for registration of existing practitioners took place in May 2000. Subsequent registrants qualify by receipt of a recognised qualification obtained from an accredited school.

The Council presently has over one-third lay membership. Under the Act, the Council is constituted as follows:

24 members made up of:

- 12 (elected) osteopath members
- 8 lay members (appointed by the Privy Council)
- 3 education members and
- 1 member appointed by the Secretary of State

Neither the 3 education members nor the Secretary of State's appointee need be osteopaths.

The General Chiropractic Council

Set up in 1998, the GCC is a United Kingdom-wide statutory body with regulatory powers, established by the Chiropractors Act 1994.

It has three main duties:

—To protect the public by establishing and operating a system of statutory regulation for chiropractors.

—To ensure the development of the profession of chiropractic, using a model of continuous improvement in practice.

—To promote the profession of chiropractic so that its contribution to the health of the nation is understood and recognised.

The General Chiropractic Council is accountable to Parliament through the Privy Council.

Council membership and appointment:

—10 chiropractors elected by registered chiropractors;

—6 members appointed by the Privy Council (must be non-chiropractors, one a medical practitioner);

—3 members appointed by the Education Committee;

—1 member appointed by the Secretary of State

There are four statutory committees:

—the Education Committee

—the Investigating Committee

—the Professional Conduct Committee

—the Health Committee

Council meetings are open to the public.

The GCC sets and publishes the Code of Practice for Chiropractors. This covers all aspects of their conduct in their dealings with patients and other health professionals. All complaints and allegations are investigated. Where a complaint is proven, the powers of the General Chiropractic Council range from a written admonishment to removing the chiropractor's name from the Register.

The GCC is financed totally from registration fees.

Source: Budd, S. & Mills, S. (2000) *Regulatory Prospects for Complementary and Alternative Medicine: Information Pack.* University of Exeter on behalf of the Department of Health

APPENDIX 3

Visit to Mr Simon Mills' CAM Practice, Department of Complementary Medicine, University of Exeter; and the Centre for Complementary Health Studies, University of Exeter
On 22/23 March 2000

Members present: Earl Baldwin of Bewdley
                        Lord Colwyn
                        Lord Haskel
                        Lord Perry of Walton
                        Lord Rea
                        Lord Soulsby of Swaffham Prior

Wednesday 22 March

Simon Mills' Clinic

On arrival at Exeter the Committee visited the clinic where Simon Mills practises. The purpose of this visit was to get a feel of a working Complementary Medicine Clinic and to meet some practising CAM therapists. The Committee were given a brief tour of the practice which consisted of: a waiting room; a small herbal medicine pharmacy where Simon Mills took questions; a treatment room where Chris Bury the clinic's osteopath demonstrated; another treatment room where Tricia Hemmingway the clinic's Alexander Technique teacher and Roger Wells a GP/psychotherapist were based; and finally the ESCOP secretariat and library.

Dinner at Crossmead Conference Centre

The Committee were welcomed by Sir Geoffrey Holland KCB, Vice Chancellor of Exeter University. Other guests at the dinner were:

Dame Margaret Turner-Warwick – Past president of the Royal College of Physicians

Professor Ruth Hawker – Chair of the local NHS trust and member of Exeter University Council

Maurice Newbound – President of the British Complementary Medicine Association

Professor Edzard Ernst – Director of the Department of Complementary Medicine and the holder of the only UK Chair in Complementary Medicine

Professor Brian Kirby – Acting Head of the Post-graduate Medical School at Exeter University

David Rogers – Head of Communications and External Relations at Exeter University

Simon Mills – Director of the Centre for Complementary Health Studies, University of Exeter

Sir Geoffrey Holland talked about Exeter University's bid to develop a new undergraduate medical school in conjunction with the University of Plymouth. The proposed curriculum for the new undergraduate medical course would include aspects of CAM. A course which promoted the awareness of other medical philosophies would be a compulsory part of the curriculum, and optional courses which explored different aspects of CAM would also be available.

Thursday 23 March

The Committee were welcomed to Senate House at the University of Exeter by Professor Brian Kirby. Professor Kirby discussed how the relationship between CAM and orthodox medicine had grown closer since he graduated 40 years ago. He also discussed how the two Exeter Departments look at both sides of complementary therapies and he highlighted the growing popularity of CAM.

Presentations by the Department for Complementary Medicine, University of Exeter

Professor Edzard Ernst

The aim of this presentation was to familiarise the Committee with the Department's work. The Department use a specific definition of CAM:

"Complementary medicine is diagnosis, treatment and/or prevention which complements mainstream medicine by contributing to a common whole, by satisfying a demand not met by orthodoxy or by diversifying the conceptual frameworks of medicine."

Ernst et al *British General Practitioner* 1995; 45:506

1. Background

The Department of Complementary Medicine was established in 1992 through a donation from the Laing Foundation, to the Centre for Complementary Health Studies (CCHS). This donation has provided a solid foundation of funding which helped establish a good infrastructure for research. In 1993 Professor Ernst was appointed Professor of Complementary Medicine and director of CCHS. In 1996 the Department of Complementary Medicine was established within the School of Postgraduate Medicine and the Directorship of CCHS was returned to Simon Mills.

The Department chose to concentrate its research on the CAM therapies that are most prevalent in the UK i.e. acupuncture, healing, herbalism, homeopathy and spinal manipulation. It also includes placebo studies. Their research aims to answer the questions: is it effective? is it safe? does it save money? The main investigative tools the Department uses are systematic reviews of published RCTs, clinical trials, surveys and other experimental studies. As well as research the Department participates in several other activities; these include the publication of FACT, holding an annual scientific meeting, occasional conferences, lectures, courses and advice.

Professor Ernst listed the strengths of the Department as: relatively strong funding, a clear focus on research, having no 'axe to grind', a staff of trained scientists, a multi-professional team, staff with 'hands on' experience with CAM treatments and numerous international collaborations, which included links with universities in the USA, Austria, Switzerland, Turkey and Germany.

2. Research into homeopathy

This part of the talk summarised some of the research that the Department has conducted into homeopathy. Several papers were discussed. The first of these was a meta-analysis (by other authors) that had looked at 89 trials of homeopathy and had concluded that the clinical effects of homeopathy were not entirely due to placebo effects. This paper had attracted a lot of attention from various medical journals. However it had also been criticised, primarily because it had examined a range of different homeopathic treatments for a range of conditions and was therefore very non–specific. In response to these criticisms a lot of further research including new analysis by Department staff has been undertaken which has looked at the effects of specific homeopathic remedies for specific complaints. These more specific studies had found no direct effect for any particular homeopathic remedy on a range of clinical problems. Research in this area at the Department is continuing.

3. General CAM Research

This part of the presentation discussed several research papers the Department has published on the perception of CAM in the UK. Professor Ernst believes that non-specific (placebo) effects are a fascinating and under-researched area which he thinks may provide a link between CAM and orthodox medicine.

One study that he described had used a questionnaire to examine levels of patient satisfaction with CAM and orthodox medicine amongst arthritis suffers who had experienced treatments by both types of practitioners. This research had found that CAM therapists were perceived as much more friendly, as having much more time to spend on the patient and the treatment, as giving more information on the treatment and on the disease, and even as giving slightly more efficacious treatments. Another study that he discussed looked at cross-referral rates between CAM and orthodox medicine and found that they were very low.

The third research area discussed was publication bias. One survey the Department had conducted had shown that CAM journals have a strong bias in favour of publishing papers which had positive results for CAM as opposed to negative or neutral results for CAM. However Professor Ernst also discussed other research which had involved submitting almost identical papers to CAM and orthodox medicine journals. The two papers both reported fictional results of an RCT that showed positive results for either a CAM therapy or an orthodox medicine therapy. They found that the paper based on an orthodox medicine treatment was more likely to be accepted for publication by an orthodox medicine journal than the identical paper which provided the same results for a CAM treatment.

Professor Ernst talked about research into the safety of CAM. He noted that the CAM community have felt that safety research is unnecessary as they feel CAM is inherently safe. He said that he felt responsible as the only UK Professor of CAM to look at safety. He discussed a survey of CAM users that had found that users could remember side effects of homeopathy, herbalism, spinal manipulation and acupuncture. However a similar survey of GPs found they could only recall having seen side effects of spinal manipulation. Later in his presentation Professor Ernst was asked whether his Department's emphasis on safety gave it a negative image in the CAM world. He answered by saying that safety is the logical first line to examine and as much of the Department's work has found in favour of the safety of CAM it should be welcomed by the CAM world. He also responded to a comment that CAM is relatively safe when compared to the levels of iatrogenic disease caused by orthodox medicine by saying that one must always keep in mind the risk/benefit balance.

The last part of this talk discussed CAM research funding which Professor Ernst described as the biggest obstacle to CAM research in the UK. A survey by the Department showed that in 1996 only 0.08% of the NHS research budget and only 0.05% of the medical charities' research budget was spent on CAM. Prof. Ernst described the CAM research funding situation in the UK as 'dismal' and compared it to the situations in Germany, the USA and Switzerland where public money is ring-fenced for CAM research. He believes that if ring fencing is done well it does not necessarily reduce the quality of research and he sees it as the only way forward. Professor Ernst also discussed what he calls the 'Catch 22' situation whereby the MRC, Wellcome Trust etc. say they would fund more CAM research if there were better research applications. He suggested that his Department's experience of rejections of grant applications has shown that the people on the research application review panels often do not understand CAM.

4. *Vision of Department's future.*

The final part of this presentation described how the Department would like to develop in the future. Professor Ernst described a Department which had an overall head of operations who was supported by a research unit, a publication unit, an education unit, an information programme and a clinical programme. The education programme would include undergraduate teaching and teaching of CAM to orthodox medicine professionals to increase communication between the two fields. The information programme would have links with journals, the media and the public and would work to counteract the misinformation present in newspapers; it would possibly be linked to NHS Direct. The clinical service would ensure that those in the unit were still seeing patients and therefore did not lose contact with those that CAM is meant to benefit, thus developing the 'ivory tower syndrome'.

Mr M. Pittler: Research into Herbal Medicinal Products

Mr Pittler started his presentation by making the point that much of CAM research is in languages other than English. He believes that one of the strengths of the Department is that they are multi-lingual and so can examine of a lot of evidence that would otherwise be inaccessible to them.

Mr Pittler discussed the prevalence of CAM in the UK. One telephone survey estimated that 20% of Britons had used CAM in the last 12 months and herbal medicine was the most likely CAM to have been used, with 34% of the share. He then discussed the top selling herbs, referring to a US survey, the results of which he suspected would be mirrored over here. This survey found that the top selling herbs were: Ginkgo, St John's Wort, Ginseng, Garlic, Echinacea, Saw Palmetto and Kava Kava (the use of which is growing very rapidly).

Research into herbal medicine can examine particular plant extracts as treatments for specific ailments so rigorous research methods can be applied. Mr. Pittler reviewed a hierarchy of evidence with systematic reviews of RCTs at the top, followed by single RCTs, controlled clinical trials and lastly uncontrolled data such as case reports which can be seen as useful in generating hypotheses. He suggested that clinical replication is important and thus he tries to concentrate on systematic reviews of RCTs which minimise selection bias, minimise random bias and can look at a range of studies and thus increase validity. However he acknowledged that such systematic reviews also have potential weaknesses in that they may include trials of poor methodological quality, they may compare non-heterogeneous data and they may reflect any existing publication bias.

The last part of this presentation reviewed specific trials the Department has carried out for specific herbs and conditions. The results of these trials showed that some herbs can be proven to be effective for certain conditions; however other herbs have, despite their popularity, produced results which are inconclusive.

Dr A. White: Research into Acupuncture

Dr White started his presentation by briefly reviewing his own background. When working as a GP in the late seventies he saw patients who were benefiting from acupuncture. At the same time the discovery of endorphins made him think that the results of acupuncture might have a rational explanation. These two events led him to train as an acupuncturist himself and when he did so he found that there was so little good quality research into acupuncture that he became a research fellow. He discussed the fact that the change from being a clinician who wanted to prove acupuncture worked, to being a researcher who had to find out whether it works or not, was a huge leap in attitude.

The rest of this presentation reviewed specific studies into the efficacy of acupuncture. None of the papers that had investigated acupuncture's efficacy had yielded conclusive or particularly positive results. He is currently involved in a study into the adverse effects of acupuncture that seems to be showing that acupuncture is relatively safe. He has also been trying to attract funding to do a study into the cost consequences of introducing CAM into primary care but has been unable to attract funding as it would be quite an expensive trial which would involve paying GPs.

Presentations by the Centre for Complementary Health Studies

Roger Hill: Introduction

Roger Hill is the programme co-ordinator and co-founder of CCHS. He provided an overview of the main features of the centre:

> The purpose of CCHS is to investigate and teach complementary health measures to practitioners. The teaching is carried out by CAM therapists.

> CCHS provides a taught MA course which covers a range of disciplines, as well as research MPhil and PhD degrees. They do not offer practical training.

> All CCHS post graduate courses emphasise research methodology which creates a tone of "mild scepticism" in all their taught modules. These modules include the therapeutic relationship, the cultural context of CAM and the holistic care of terminally ill patients.

> They welcome those who practise orthodox medicine disciplines as well as CAM ones as they acknowledge there is much to learn from orthodox medicine although they object to medical imperialism.

> CCHS has links with Bristol Cancer Help Centre and the Thomas Jefferson University in the USA.

> CCHS will soon become part of the Department of Lifelong Learning at Exeter University.

Roger Hill aired some concern about the growth of generic undergraduate courses in complementary health studies which offer a smattering of knowledge about a range of disciplines. He suggested these should not be seen to qualify graduates to practise and that the organisations (often umbrella bodies) who support such courses are of variable reliability.

Sarah Budd: Department of Health Scoping Study

In 1999 the Department of Health commissioned CCHS to produce an information pack reviewing the process of regulation, to pilot a standards validation mechanism and to update the 1997 study which surveyed all the CAM professional organisations in the UK. Sarah Budd's presentation launched the updated version of this study which is the main reference document describing CAM organisations in the UK and includes contact details for all the bodies surveyed. The 1997 report had recommended integrative moves in all CAM fields; this second study inquired about the progress organisations had made towards integration.

The main demographic findings of the new survey were:

> There are approximately 50,000 CAM practitioners in the UK, some of whom are members of more than one organisation.

> There are approximately 10,000 statutory health professionals who practise some form of CAM.

> Up to 5 million patients have consulted a CAM practitioner in the last year.

True figures are difficult to ascertain as many practitioners will not be members of any organisation, and some organisations will not have responded to the survey.

Despite the desire for greater integration expressed in the last report and generally encouraging movement since, there was in fact some evidence of greater diversification. The report contains a section on emerging and complex organisations and a pilot study of the processes involved in improving co-ordination within on therapy (reflexology).

Sarah Budd highlighted the fact that over the last two years regulation has become one of the main concerns for CAM.

Mr M. Willoughby: Herbal Standards

CCHS has been working in collaboration with the British Herbal Medical Association to produce quality standards for herbal medicines. The CCHS received a large grant from the European Union in 1994 to support various efforts. These include:

- Overcoming problems which arise because many herbs, once processed, look the same. Different products can be identified using thin layer chromatography and microscopy. Results from this work have been collected together in the British Herbal Pharmacopeia for manufacturers to use as reference material.

- Producing the Phytonet web-site for information about herbal medicine. This web-site includes a reporting system for any adverse effects.

- Producing ESCOP monographs on the medicinal uses of plant drugs. These monographs use the 'core SPC' (Summary Product Characteristics) format and are being considered by the European Medicines Evaluation Agency for use in assessing licensing applications across Europe.

Mr M. Bovey: Acupuncture Resource Research Centre

Mr Bovey began his presentation by describing his work running the Acupuncture Resource Research Centre. The centre was set up in 1994 by the British Acupuncture Council, and is wholly funded by them; it promotes acupuncture generally and encourages research mindedness. In order to do this the Centre:

Responds to requests

Provides direct support for practitioners

Interprets research by producing briefing papers

Supports other research groups by giving lectures, hosting symposiums etc.

Supplies a purpose built data base and literature searches for treating patients with unusual conditions.

Professor B. Goodwin: Academic Challenges

Professor Goodwin is a professor of biology and was first external examiner for CCHS. He currently teaches a module at the Centre which attempts to bring together alternative and conventional theories of health. The part of the module he discussed in this talk concerned complexity theory and health.

Student Presentations

In order to give an idea of the diverse work of the CCHS, several students gave brief presentations on the progress of their studies at the Centre. These were:

Lizzie Baines — an MA candidate who also works as a specialist palliative care nurse. She discussed her dissertation : 'An audit of Tibetan medical practice in the UK.'

Helen Cooke — an MA candidate who also works as the therapy director for Bristol Cancer Help Centre and is a registered nurse. She discussed her dissertation: 'An evaluation of the role of the Bristol Cancer Help Centre in helping patients and their supporters through its advice on complementary therapies and self -help techniques.

Reg d'Souza — a BPhil graduate who works as a physiotherapist and an acupuncturist. He discussed his dissertation: ' Trigger point acupuncture and ultrasonic therapy in low back pain.'

Penny Franklin — an MA candidate who also works as a health visitor and a nurse. She discussed her dissertation: 'Parental perceptions of the effects of lack of sleep on the couple relationship of parents with children between the ages of 12 and 30 months.'

Jessie Ng Fong Tiao — an MA graduate who works as a nurse, an acupuncturist and a Chinese herbalist. She discussed her dissertation: 'A single blind, cross-over study to measure the effect of acupuncture on low back pain.'

Ian Oliver — an MPhil candidate who also works as a homeopath. He discussed his dissertation: 'The homeopathic treatment of benign breast tumours.'

Vicki Pitman — an MPhil graduate who works as a medical herbalist. She discussed her dissertation: ' The relationship between ancient Greek and Ayurvedic medicine.'

Bridget Simpson — an MA graduate who works as a dental surgeon. She discussed her dissertation: 'An investigation into 'dry socket': a pilot study of a new herbal treatment.'

Frances Turner — an MPhil candidate who also works as an acupuncturist and Chinese herbalist. She discussed her dissertation: ' An evaluation of whether some form of standardisation of the English vocabulary of Chinese medicine would raise the standards of understanding and practice of Chinese medicine in the UK.'

Tina Wong — an MA and PhD graduate who also works as an acupuncturist, a nurse and a midwife. She discussed her dissertation: 'The use of traditional medicine and rituals in the prevention and treatment of post-natal depression among the Kadazan/Dasan and Bajan/Malay communities of East Malaysia.'

APPENDIX 4

Visit to the Marylebone Health Centre, 12 April 2000

Members present: Earl Baldwin of Bewdley
                        Lord Colwyn
                        Lord Perry of Walton
                        Lord Rea
                        Lord Walton of Detchant (Chairman)

On arrival at the Health Centre the members of the Sub-Committee were welcomed by the staff, who included:

                        Dr Tania Eber — GP
                        Martin Gerish — practice manager
                        Dr Goodstone — GP
                        Gerry Harris — acupuncturist
                        Chrissie Melhuish — massage therapist
                        Dr Sue Morrison — GP
                        Dr Richard Morrison — GP
                        Dr David Peters — osteopath
                        Gabrielle Pinto — homeopath

Dr Sue Morrison described Marylebone Health Centre (MHC). The health centre was started 12 years ago by Dr Patrick Pietroni and Dr Derek Chase. The original objective was to "*explore and evaluate ways in which primary healthcare can be delivered to a deprived area in addition to the General Practice component. The approach is to include an holistic component comprising an education self-help model and a complementary healthcare model.*"

The primary focus of the practice is collaboration with many types of healthcare professionals including complementary therapists. There is also a focus on internal collaboration with patients and a big issue for the practice is power sharing; there is a patient partnership group and patients are involved in the strategy forming group. The practice aims to be a model that can be useful in other NHS centres.

MHC has a local catchment area like any other NHS practice and it does not offer private treatment. To access CAM services, patients must be referred by one of the GPs at the practice. It has been found that some patients register purely to get access to CAM, and this is discouraged as it is thought preferable for the patient to have built up a relationship with a GP before in-house referral. The demographics of the patients of the practice are characteristic of an inner city GP practice. However it is a very mobile population due to a high proportion of students, homeless people and political refugees. The practice has a high turnover rate of 50% per annum.

Introduction to Integrative Approaches - David Peters.

David Peters discussed research at the centre. MHC is a multidisciplinary practice with an emphasis on inter-professional learning. It is linked to the University of Westminster Centre for Community Care and Primary Health, which is interested in integrating relevant aspects of complementary therapy appropriately into multi-disciplinary mainstream NHS Care. He explained that the two organisations work together and that, in a sense, MHC is laboratory of the university.

He discussed how integrated medicine is an emerging field and that therefore they had had to develop intuitively in response to patients' and practitioners' needs. However, their research has also had to try and address the Cochrane Questions such as: Can it work? Does it work in practice and Is it worth it? He explained that one of the challenges in the area of integrated medicine is that it is about more than just combining orthodox medicine and CAM therapies, it is about emphasising health promotion and self-care and about collaboration between practitioners and developing the practitioner-patient relationship.

He discussed the history of research at MHC. Between 1987-1992 the Centre was part of the St Mary's-Waites project and the main questions they were looking at were whether integrated healthcare had a role in primary health, and whether it was an acceptable and appropriate area to encourage. In the 90s they have moved on to investigating the best methods for integrated delivery. Now (under a new grant) they are looking at specific intake criteria and outcome measures. These changes in research focus have been developing at the same time as a change in UK medical attitudes towards CAM, which he summarised as having gone from the idea of CAM as fringe, to alternative, to complementary and now to integrated.

Dr Peters described the six stages of integrating CAM into general practice and discussed the main questions to be tackled at each stage. These were:

1) Practice review - what needs are being poorly met?
2) Resource assessment - is CAM relevant? what is its evidence base? is integration feasible?
3) Designing a service - asking how will GPs use the service? what will be its aims? how will complementary practitioners be integrated into the primary care team?
4) Delivering the service - developing referral procedures and working on resource monitoring.
5) Management servicing – including quality assurance procedures and evaluating outcomes,
6) Modifying the service in response to experience.

Once modification has taken place the steps can start all over again, so the service is constantly self-monitoring and improving.

Dr Peters discussed the question of how to decide when GPs should consider a CAM referral. At MHC it was decided to do this only for conditions where some evidence for efficacy of a particular CAM existed. It was also decided referrals would only take place if GPs wanted to refer, and complementary practitioners thought they could help and had an interest in helping. They have now developed a list of conditions that they commonly consider for CAM referrals. These included complex chronic illnesses such as chronic fatigue syndrome; stress-related conditions; asthma; IBS; eczema and allergies; migraine. GPs consider a referral if there is a new diagnosis of one of these conditions and one of the following criteria applies: (a)r orthodox medicine has failed; (b) the patient is suffering side-effects from the orthodox medicine; (c) the patient requests CAM for one of these conditions; or (d) if the GP feels it is a complex case where CAM may help (and having asked the CAM therapist they, too, feel they may be able to help.)

Dr Peters finished his talk by describing how research has the capacity to serve both practitioners' and patients' needs. For example, audit ensures quality assurance, research through qualitative methods increases understanding of the patient's experience, action research promotes service and professional development and case studies illustrate best practice models. In this way practice-based research promotes quality and understanding.

Demonstration of Use of IT System for Quality Assurance Audit - Gerry Harris

Gerry Harris, an acupuncturist at the practice, demonstrated how patients are referred to complementary therapists at the practice, and how the complementary therapists record the progress of their treatment package in a way that makes clinical audit possible.

Patients at the practice can only see complementary practitioners if they are referred by one of the GPs. The practice has two forms for such referrals - one with the basic referral information and the other a Measure Your Own Medical Outcome Profile (MYMOP). The MYMOP form describes what each patient's primary and secondary (and if applicable subsequent) complaints are and the patient has to rate how much they are suffering. The information from the MYMOP is put on a specially designed computer programme. Each time the patient goes to their complementary therapist they rate how they are feeling and this is entered into the computer with other relevant information. This creates a log of the progress of the referral and the computer generates graphs logging improvement (or lack of it) in each patient.

Demonstration of Complementary Therapies.

The Members of the sub-committee were invited to watch patients being treated by one of the complementary therapists present. The demonstrations provided were:

Massage Therapy

Chrissie Melhuish, a massage therapist, treated a patient with whiplash complicated by sports injuries and chronic stress. The practitioner was a trained nurse, with experience of both osteopathy and sports medicine. She described her approach to patients with stress-related problems: long sessions (1 hour), with time to talk; and self-help, involving exercises and stress-management techniques. She expressed doubt whether the ITEC qualification was adequate in itself for safe practice.

Homeopathy

Gabrielle Pinto, a homeopath, treated a patient with a history of Irritable Bowel Syndrome and panic attacks. The practitioner had being seeing the patient for about 18 months. She explained that the first few sessions with a patient usually involves finding the right remedy for that patient and this may take a while. If the patient is taking a lot of orthodox medical drugs, she often starts by recommending herbal medicines before moving onto homeopathic remedies. Once the right therapy is found patients can often self-medicate at home, but if they have relapses or need high-potency remedies they come back to see the homeopath. The patient present at this demonstration reported improvement with both her complaints and she attributed this to homeopathy. She claimed her homeopathic treatment has allowed her to stop being reliant on the drugs her GP had been prescribing, which had included Colepermin and Beta-Blockers. She also felt she did not need to visit GPs so often now she was seeing the homeopath. When asked if she would have gone to a homeopath herself if she had not been referred on the NHS, she said she would have if she could have found an affordable one but that would have been unlikely.

Acupuncture

Gerry Harris, an acupuncturist, treated a patient with multiple problems (including leukaemia) for which she was also receiving orthodox treatment. The patient felt the acupuncture helped to 'keep her balanced' throughout her illness. Gerry Harris described how she leaves the needles in patients for about 20 minutes and therefore if two treatment rooms are available she can treat two patients at once, thus improving her treatment rate.

Meeting with Practitioners and Patients

The Sub-Committee were introduced to seven patients who had received complementary therapies at the Centre, many of whom were members of the patient-partnership association. Each of these patients had suffered from very different complaints including asthma, back pain (following a car accident where vertebrae were broken), cancer, recurrent urinary tract infections and chronic rhinitis. All the patients had tried a variety of orthodox treatments before being referred to complementary therapists at the practice, and all felt that they had benefited from CAM. Many claimed it had reduced their reliance on the orthodox medicine they were using before referral

Evidence-based Practice – David Peters

David Peters discussed the applicability research to real-life practice. He suggested that, although RCTs and meta-analysis of RCTs are valuable, in that they provide certainty about the efficacy of a medication for a particular condition, real-life primary care does not mirror the way illness and treatment are defined in such research. He explained patients do not come to their GPs with specific, well-defined conditions but the intake for most trials eliminates all but the most clear-cut examples of a condition. He suggested that this was especially a problem for CAM as the GPs often referred the more complicated patients who had chronic complex conditions. Often these patients were not suffering from a single problem, although a particular condition may have been the reason for referral but further discussion often unveiled other problems.

He also discussed the problem of how to shape outcome criteria for research into CAM. The complementary therapists at the practice had considered a number of instruments for evaluating outcome. These included questionnaires such as the SF36. However, many of these instruments required a lot of time and thought from the patients so the MHC had decided to opt for the MYMOP form. They are piloting this form but say that using any standard instrument is hard as they get such a variety of patients.

In summary David Peters suggested that a variety of research methods should be used for CAM. RCTs should be used as they have a high standard of rigour but outcomes research can complement RCTs and can be designed in a way that has more relevance to primary care. Together he believes it is possible to build an evidence 'mosaic'. They are making efforts to create their own research, and early results show that many patients are doing well. Dr Peters feels that it is possible to create rigorous data within a patient-centred practice with vague entry criteria. Their eventual aim is more rigour in their research methods, for example through randomising patients to different treatments.

Practice-based Evidence – Dr Sue Morrison

Dr Sue Morrison started her talk by saying that the issues of evidence-based practice and practice-based evidence were related.

She moved on to describe the status of the practice which is a PMS Pilot, and therefore it is on a devolved budget. However Dr Morrison suggested that their PCG is moving towards a PMS-type structure and if they had known this was going to happen then they may not have taken up the offer of the PMS Pilot.

Although their status on the PMS pilot means that MHC is different from the rest of their local PCG, they are trying to stay integrated. Dr Morrison herself is on the board of a sub-group of the PCG that is looking into opening up CAM provision to the whole of the PCG. This plan is currently only in development but they have decided that GPs and complementary practitioners will only be able to refer into the service if they have been on a course about integration which is being developed.

Dr Morrison explained that as a practice they have always been in favour of rigorous clinical audit and they are using data from their audits to develop a manual of integrated care for other practices to use. However she described some limitations to their data, such as the fact that some patients self-select to MHC in order to access CAM, and therefore wider information is needed from across the PCG on what patients want.

She finished her talk by saying that although the practice has been dutiful to NHS policy they are also hoping to be able to inform it.

Discussion

Many questions about research were discussed. These included points on the problem of how to randomise for time spent with patients, and how to take account of a variety of possible confounding factors such as whether a patient pays for the service and how this may affect their reaction to a treatment. One point that was emphasised was that research involving CAM must ensure that the CAM practitioners involved are properly trained as there is a mix of training standards in the area. The staff at MHC are talking about developing a research management group to tackle such issues. However some worries were aired that the future of services like those provided at MHC may be in danger during the first few years of PCGs when money is tight, and those in management are anxious and have a big enough task just managing orthodox medical services.

APPENDIX 5

Visit to the University of Southampton Medical School and the Centre for the Study of Complementary Medicine, Southampton, on 9 June 2000

Members present: Earl Baldwin of Bewdley
                                     Lord Haskel
                                     Lord Rea
                                     Lord Tombs
                                     Lord Walton of Detchant

Complementary Medicine Research Unit: School of Medicine, University of Southampton.

Professor Arthur, Head of School of Medicine

Professor Arthur, Head of the School of Medicine, welcomed the Committee and explained that the research structure was developed 'from the ground up' from 1990. Their research concentrates on areas of expertise which are: human genetics; infection, inflammation and repair; cancer services; foetal origins of adult disease; and community clinical services. The medical school is the second smallest in the country but was rated in the top ten in the research assessment exercise and scored well in the quality assessment exercise.

Dr George Lewith

Dr George Lewith, doctor, researcher and CAM practitioner, discussed his work as Head of the Complementary Medicine Research Unit where he works for half a day per week. The unit was set up in 1995 and is situated within the infection, inflammation and repair unit of the research division of the medical school. The unit is financed by 'soft money' rather than by the medical school. Its main funding source is a grant from the Laing Foundation (which also funded much of the work the Committee saw at Exeter), which has covered all their administrative costs since May 1995 to May 1998 with a further three years support promised until May 2001. They have also received money for research from the Wellcome Trust and the British Medical Association as well as some money from industry for commercial research.

The aim of the research unit is to evaluate the clinical effects of complementary medicine and investigate the scientific basis for its mechanisms. They believe that 'these innovative techniques should be rigorously assessed and, where appropriate, integrated into mainstream conventional medicine.'

The research that they do falls into five main headings: rheumatology and rehabilitation work, respiratory disease, cancer, fundamental research (including health psychology and research on the effects of attitudes on outcomes), chronic fatigue syndrome and miscellaneous projects.

Dr Lewith highlighted some of the lessons that they had learnt in their work at the unit. Firstly, large, good quality clinical trials can help uncover information that even people working as practitioners had not thought about. Secondly, having a CAM research unit within an undergraduate medical school provides a clear research structure as well as administrative and research support, and working in an NHS environment provides access to patients as well as providing credibility for the unit. Thirdly, designing and carrying out rigorous trials in CAM is more intellectually challenging than orthodox medicine research: it can be done but it is not easy. Dr Lewith's final point was that setting up a research unit and carrying out good quality research in the CAM area takes a long time. They found that it took four to five years of hard work before they had good quality, interesting papers coming through.

Overview of various trials

The next set of presentations was given by some researchers and students who worked within the unit. Dr Lewith said the Unit had made an effort to show a cross section of studies including ones with positive and negative results and ones in progress as well as ones completed. The studies included work into acupuncture for chronic neck pain, work on the relationship between patients' attitudes to CAM and the outcomes of their treatment, the proving of Belladonna in homeopathic dilutions, electrodermal testing for allergies and acupuncture in stroke rehabilitation.

Questions

When asked if the level of funding the unit got from its NHS region was unusual, George Lewith said it was but he believed part of the reason for this is that they submit unusually high-quality proposals and they take account of any criticisms their proposals receive during peer review and re-submit accordingly. He also mentioned that NHS review can be useful even if the NHS region can not afford to fund the project. If the NHS peer review says it is a good quality proposal, the Unit can use that recommendation to get support from charities which are too small to have their own peer review panels but want validation of a proposal before they fund it.

However Professor Arthur noted that Southampton has recently changed NHS regions from the South West to the South East region and since this change they have noticed a drop in medical school funding (not just for CAM proposals) because the South East is a more competitive region.

Education

Dr Chris Stevens gave a brief overview of the medical school curriculum. It is a five year undergraduate course with optional modules (one option being in CAM) available in year three and an in-depth research study unit in year four. In year five students take up placements across the region.

Dr David Owen, a local homeopathic physician and President of the Faculty of Homeopathy, is the course tutor for the CAM module. This covers eight half days and is a familiarisation course, not a training one. It covers questions such as: which therapies can be used for which conditions? and, what is CAM appropriate and inappropriate for? The main therapies the students come into contact with, and consider evidence about, are acupuncture, homeopathy, chiropractic, osteopathy and herbal medicine.

Dr Owen said the course is centred around the question: "If you had a loved one who was suffering from an illness not well treated by orthodox medicine, what would you want their doctor to know about CAM?" The course involves complementary practitioners in the local area and offers medical students an opportunity to experience CAM as practised in the community. The course is in great demand, with numbers limited by places, not by the amount of interest shown by students.

The learning objectives for the course have been developed by the teaching team, with input from medical students studying the module:

- To have examined (constructively and critically) the merits and claims of different complementary medicines.

- To describe the concepts of individualisation and holism, and to give examples of when different CAM treatment approaches are used to treat different patients with the same diagnosis.

- To have examined the students' own attitudes towards complementary medicine and reflect on the variety of attitudes that exist among patients, health care practitioners and providers.

- To be able to assess and advise patients who enquire about or benefit from CAM.

- To have participated in consultations and discussions to identify how patients perceive different treatment approaches and the role patients play in healing themselves.

- To state the basic principles and evidence for complementary medicine. To describe the context in which it is practised in the community and how to obtain more information, including key points on training and regulation.

Dr Owen also outlined some issues that had arisen when deciding how to design the course. These included:

- Which CAM therapies to teach

- Whether to include clinical attachments

- How to develop common objectives with courses at other medical schools

- What methods to use in assessment

- Limitations of the module structure

- Funding

- Post graduate teaching

Other healthcare practitioners training at Southampton (e.g. nurses) can attend the course as can students from the Bournemouth College of Chiropractic who may want to learn about other CAM therapies. This encourages interdisciplinary learning and understanding.

Aside from the CAM module several of the medical students have been involved with the unit through pilot research projects on CAM issues during the research part of their course in the fourth year). The medical school also runs lectures in the second year of the curriculum on acupuncture and pain management.

Dr Owen also mentioned his work outside Southampton. He has done some work on Continuing Professional Development in CAM for doctors; he has found the postgraduate course in homeopathy at the Glasgow Homeopathic Hospital is the most popular postgraduate course for doctors in Scotland.

Centre for the Study of Complementary Medicine

Introduction and Background

After lunch the Committee visited the centre for the Study of Complementary Medicine where they were welcomed by Jacqueline Tuson, Practice Manager. She introduced the other members of staff who included:

- Dr George Lewith - GP, CAM practitioner and joint partner in the centre

- Dr Michael Clerk - GP, CAM practitioner and joint partner.

- Maureen Middleton - Nurse manager

- Val Hopwood - Physiotherapist, CAM practitioner and researcher

- Alan Mills - practitioner

Ms Tuson described the background of the Centre. The Centre was set up in 1982 by Dr Lewith and a Dr Kenyon. The partners are all medically qualified practitioners who previously worked as orthodox GPs and hospital doctors. They also use a range of qualified CAM practitioners alongside the partners to complete the range of therapies they can offer. They have built up their reputation so that they now have 4000 patients on their current database and the doctors see up to 20 patients a day from across the British Isles and Europe. They also have a smaller sister clinic in Upper Harley Street.

The conventional medical background of the doctors and practitioners is an important element to the Centre as it gives the public confidence in their abilities and improves relationships with local GPs, resulting in more referrals. It is also important that all the practitioners are multi-skilled and are not limited to the use of one CAM therapy so that they often use a mixture of therapies in one treatment plan.

They have their own dispensary and qualified nurses who provide advice and support for patients. This is part of the Centres emphasis on a team based approach. They have a nurse advice line for patients with worries as well as a web-site with information on treatments.

The fact that they have the phrase 'for the study of' in their title means they get numerous phone calls from people who do not realise they are a clinical practise. The reason they keep this title is because historically they did a great deal of training and research from the Centre. However they do not currently offer training courses but they keep their title because providing information is part of their mission.

A survey of the Centre which was published in the BMJ shows most patients come with very long term problems (average duration 10 years). Currently patients most frequently present with the following conditions: irritable bowel syndrome, migraine, eczema, non-specific allergy, back pain and chronic fatigue. The staff continuously audit their practice, and results for 1999 show impressive outcomes for a lot of patients suffering from chronic conditions such as IBS and ME.

The Dorset NHS Contract

The Centre for the Study of Complementary Medicine is primarily a private practice but it has a history of providing NHS care too. Until recently this was provided under the fund-holding scheme for local fund-holding practices. Other practices in the area were able to refer patients through the Health Authority, and these patients had to meet stringent criteria. This system led to a difference in availability between those practices which were fund-holding and those which were not. The abolition of fund-holding has meant that patients in the Southampton area can usually obtain referral to the Centre if their GP thinks it would be the best treatment for them.

As well as their relationship with the local PCGs the Centre has a separate NHS agreement with the Dorset Area Health Authority. This is a unique contract within the NHS for CAM services. It operates in two parts. The first is an integrated medicine unit which operates for one day per month at a GP practice in Dorset. GPs in this clinic and in other local clinics are able to refer patients with any of six specific conditions to this clinic. These conditions are: chronic fatigue syndrome, IBS, migraine, child behavioural problems, eczema and non specific allergy. There is a waiting list of around three months for this clinic; at times this has been as long as nine months. Prescriptions are limited to what is available on the NHS unless patients are willing to pay for medicines themselves.

The second contract with the Dorset Area Health Authority allows patients to travel to the Centre in Southampton for their treatment. Last year this resulted in 600 consultations. This system provides for the same six conditions as the first contract although there is some flexibility. This service is quite popular with GPs as they can send patients who are difficult and who they have been unable to help. This is a more comprehensive contract as the range of treatments they can provide at the Centre is greater and the nurses and dispensary can be used. The contract is very easy to administer as it provides for 6 appointments for the specified condition with the only formality being a letter of referral. The contract also requires a letter of progress be sent to the referring GP. The six appointments can be extended if the GP writes to the Health Authority for permission. The Centre makes a conscious effort to make sure GPs are always kept up to date about their patients' progress and treatment. This contract has allowed interested GPs to become fully informed about the Centre's methods and they see this as being of long term benefit to the NHS.

Case Studies

The Committee were then introduced to a patient who had received treatment at the Centre and had the opportunity to ask questions about how they had viewed their treatment and what they felt about their experiences.

Therapeutic Demonstrations

The Committee were given the opportunity to participate in or watch demonstrations of the Alexander Technique and Acupuncture, and to ask questions of the practitioners involved.

APPENDIX 6

*Special visit to the Glasgow Homeopathic Hospital by two members of the Sub-Committee
on 24 August 2000*

Members present: Lord Perry of Walton
                    Lord Walton of Detchant

The Homeopathic Hospital is in the grounds of the Gartnavel General Hospital in the west of Glasgow. The building, which is extremely attractive, is owned by the NHS but the capital costs needed to erect the building were all obtained from private sources. There is an in-patient unit of 14 beds, with extensive out-patient facilities, and access to all of the more sophisticated radiological and other investigative activities of the General Hospital nearby. Some 400 patients are admitted to the unit annually. All out-patients are seen by reference from general practitioners or medical consultants in Glasgow. One great advantage is that the doctors are not, as a rule, required to see more than one, or at the most two, new patients in a single out-patient session, so that there is ample time for full and detailed consultation; this enables them to practise "whole patient" or so-called holistic medicine. Medical students are regularly attached to the Homeopathic Hospital on an elective basis.

Homeopathic remedies of all types are widely employed but whenever appropriate, and particularly in serious disease, conventional medical treatment is provided. In essence, therefore, the unit practises integrated medicine.

A detailed discussion took place about the research of the unit with Dr David Reilly and with the Unit Manager and two of Dr Reilly's colleagues, one a consultant, like him, in general internal medicine, and the other an associate specialist. Dr Reilly pointed out that they have great difficulty in raising funds for research, though they have obtained some from private sources and some through NHS mechanisms.

Discussions ranged widely over the role of homeopathic medicine and the mechanism of action of homeopathic remedies. Dr Reilly agreed that many biochemists find the concept of homeopathic treatment puzzling and difficult to accept, but pointed out that in his opinion the biophysicists had much less difficulty in understanding the validity of the mechanism by which homeopathic remedies may act.

APPENDIX 7

Sub-Committee 1

The members of the Sub-Committee which conducted this Inquiry were:

Earl Baldwin of Bewdley (co-opted)
Lord Colwyn (co-opted)
Lord Haskel
Lord Howie of Troon
Lord Perry of Walton
Lord Quirk
Lord Rea
Lord Smith of Clifton (co-opted)
Lord Soulsby of Swaffham Prior (co-opted)
Lord Tombs
Lord Walton of Detchant (Chairman)

The Sub-Committee had as its specialist advisers Professor Stephen Holgate, Clinical Professor of Immunopharmacology, University of Southampton, and Mr Simon Mills, Director of the Centre for Complementary Health Studies, University of Exeter.

Members declared the following interests in relation to this Inquiry:

Earl Baldwin of Bewdley— Joint Chairman of the Parliamentary Group on Alternative and Complementary Medicine; patron of the Natural Medicines Society; patron of the National Federation of Spiritual Healers.

Lord Colwyn— President of the Parliamentary Group on Alternative and Complementary Medicine; President, Natural Medicines Society; President, Arterial Health Foundation; patron of the Research Council for Complementary Medicine; patron of the Blackie Foundation; patron of the Foundation for Traditional Chinese Medicines; patron of the National Federation of Spiritual Healers; Council Member of the Medical Protection Society; Chairman, Dental Protection Ltd; member of the Royal Society of Medicine.

Lord Rea — Former NHS general practitioner; former lecturer in Social (Public Health) Medicine at St Thomas's Hospital Medical School; Fellow of the Royal Society of Medicine (former President of Section of General Practice); Hon. Secretary of National Heart Forum (former Vice-Chairman); Chairman of All-Party Parliamentary Food and Health Forum; Treasurer of All-Party Parliamentary Group on Drug Abuse; Trustee of Action Research; Medicinal Cannabis Foundation; Patron of Connect Foundation for Mental Health; Vice-Patron of Child Psychotherapy Trust, MIND.

Lord Soulsby of Swaffham Prior— President, Royal Society of Medicine (until 18 July 2000); member of a committee which advises the British Veterinary Association on, among other things, alternative medicines and practices.

Lord Tombs— Chairman, Goldsmiths Education Committee, which sponsors courses for A-level science teachers, including a course on complementary and alternative medicine.

Lord Walton of Detchant— Former Professor of Neurology and Dean of Medicine, University of Newcastle upon Tyne; former Warden, Green College, University of Oxford; former President, British Medical Association, Royal Society of Medicine, General Medical Council, Association of British Neurologists and World Federation of Neurology; occasional neuroscience adviser to a pharmaceutical company; patron, Action for Disability, International Spinal Research Trust, National Head Injuries Association (Headway), North Northumberland Day Hospice, Oxford International Biomedical Centre, 'Puff-In' Appeal (cystic fibrosis), Radcliffe Medical Foundation; Vice-Patron, Brendoncare Foundation; President, Hampra, Neurosciences Research Foundation; Vice-

President, Epilepsy Research Foundation, Guideposts Trust; Life President, Muscular Dystrophy Group of Great Britain and Northern Ireland; member of the King's Fund Working Party on Osteopathy and Chiropractic.

Lord Winston—

Practising medical academic, occasionally using complementary techniques — particularly acupuncture — for patients. Currently conducting a trial of the effect of trace elements on human fertility and miscarriage.

APPENDIX 8

List of Witnesses

The following witnesses gave evidence. Those marked * gave oral evidence.

* Academy of Medical Royal Colleges (Royal College of Anaesthetists Pain Management Committee and Royal College of Physicians)
* Academy of Medical Sciences
  Academy of On-Site Massage
  Acupuncture Association of Chartered Physiotherapists
  Advertising Standards Authority
  Alpha Omega Resources Ltd
  Aromatherapy Trade Council and Aromatherapy Organisations Council
  Association of British Insurers
* Association of British Veterinary Acupuncturists
  Association of Light Touch Therapists
* Association of Medical Research Charities
  Association of Reflexologists
  Australian Department of Health, Therapeutic Goods Administration
  Ayurvedic Medical Association UK
  BHA Hypnotherapy Association
  Professor Michael Baum
  Lucy Bell
  Dr Susan Blackmore
  Boston College
  Breast UK
* Dr Thurstan Brewin (HealthWatch)
  Bristol Cancer Help Centre
  British Academy of Western Acupuncture
* British Acupuncture Council
  British Chiropractic Association
  British College of Naturopathy and Osteopathy
* British Complementary Medicine Association
* British Dental Association
  British Embassy, Beijing
  British Embassy, Washington
  British Holistic Medical Association
* British Homoeopathic Dental Association
  British Library
* British Medical Acupuncture Society
* British Medical Association
  British Medical Hypnotherapy Examinations Board
  British Naturopathic Association
  British Pharmacological Society
  British School of Osteopathy
* British Society for Allergy Environmental and Nutritional Medicine
  British Society of Medical and Dental Hypnosis
  Sarah Budd
  BUPA Hospitals Ltd
  Cavendish Centre for Cancer Care
  Centre for the Study of Complementary Medicine
  Professor Kelvin Chan
  Chinese Herbal Medicine & Health Care Ltd
  Chinese Medicine Association of Suppliers
  Wainwright Churchill
  College of Chiropractors
* Commission for Health Improvement
* Committee on Safety of Medicines
  Commonwealth Working Group on Traditional and Complementary Health Systems
  Complementary Medical Services for Prisoners
* Consumers' Association
  Consumers for Health Choice
  Ivan Corea, Fellow, King's Fund

Corporation of Advanced Hypnotherapy
* Council of Heads of Medical Schools and Committee of Vice Chancellors
    and Principals
Council for Professions Supplementary to Medicine
Alison Denham
Doctor-Healer Network
John Dudderidge
Eastern Medicine (Tibb) Practitioners Association
Audrey Edwards
* European Agency for the Evaluation of Medicinal Products
* European Herbal Practitioners Association
* European Scientific Cooperative on Phytotherapy
* Faculty of Homeopathy, Homeopathic Trust and British Homoeopathic
    Association
Federation of Clinical Shiatsu Practitioners
Foresight fertility clinic
Foundation for Conductive Education
* Foundation for Integrated Medicine
Foundation for Traditional Chinese Medicine
Richard Fuller
* General Chiropractic Council
* General Dental Council
* General Medical Council
* General Osteopathic Council
Dr John Gibson
Dr Norman Gourlay
Dr Andrew Griffiths
Wendy Grossman, *Skeptic* Magazine
Harley Street Clinic
Haven Trust
* Department of Health
Health Food Manufacturers' Association
* HealthWatch
* Healthwork UK
Homeopathic Medical Association
Lorraine Horton
Hypnotherapy Society
IBIS International Corporation
Independent Healthcare Association
Institute of Biology, British Association for Lung Research, British
    Electrophoresis Society and British Association for Psychopharmacology
Institute of Postgraduate Studies (transcendental meditation)
Integrated Medicine Group
International Federation of Reflexologists
Institute for Complementary Medicine, British General Council of
    Complementary Medicine, British Register of Complementary Practitioners
International Society of Professional Aromatherapists
Dennis Ives
Timothy Jackson and Jacky Owens
Kesteven Natural Health Centre
Kinesiology National Occupational Standard Association Steering Group
* Linda Lazarides (Nutritional Therapy Council)
Mrs Ann Lett
Alan Lettin
Dr George Lewith, University of Southampton School of Medicine
Maharishi Foundation
Dr Peter Mansfield
* Medical Research Council
Middlesex University Chinese Medicine Ethics Committee
Ian Miller
NHS Alliance
NHS Centre for Reviews and Dissemination, University of York
NHS Confederation

Napier University, Edinburgh
National Association of Health Stores
* National Federation of Spiritual Healers
* National Institute for Clinical Excellence
National Office of Animal Health
* Natural Medicines Society
A Nelson & Co Ltd
* Roger Newman Turner
Valerie Nicholson
* Nutritional Therapy Council
Parliamentary Group for Alternative and Complementary Medicine
Patient Concern
* Patients' Association
Dr Anne Pettigrew
Prevention of Professional Abuse Network
Professional Association of Alexander Teachers
* Proprietary Association of Great Britain
Radionic Association
Radionic and Radiesthesia Trust
Register of Chinese Herbal Medicine
* Research Council for Complementary Medicine
David Leslie Robinson
Royal Free and University College Medical School
* Royal College of General Practitioners
* Royal College of Nursing
Royal College of Obstetricians and Gynaecologists
Royal College of Paediatrics and Child Health
Royal College of Physicians of Edinburgh
Royal College of Psychiatrists
Royal College of Veterinary Surgeons
Royal London Homoeopathic Hospital
* Royal Pharmaceutical Society
* Royal Society
Royal Society of Edinburgh
Sailing with Spirit
Adrian Seager
Shiatsu Society UK
Shiatsu International
Harry Simpson
* Society of Homoeopaths
Society of Teachers of the Alexander Technique
Julie Stone
* Dr Stephen Straus, National Center for Complementary and Alternative
     Medicine, Maryland, USA
Thrive
Tibbi Naturopathic Medical Foundation
Dr Richard Tonkin
David Tredinnick MP
UK Cochrane Centre
* UK Central Council for Nursing, Midwifery and Health Visiting
University of Central Lancashire Faculty of Health
University of Exeter School of Postgraduate Medicine and Health Sciences
University of Oxford Faculty of Clinical Medicine
University of Surrey School of Biological Sciences
University of Wales Institute, Cardiff
University of Westminster Centre for Community Care and Primary Health
Vedic Medical Hall Ltd
Dr Alan Watkins, Hunter Kane Resource Management
* Wellcome Trust
Dr Midge Whitelegg
Raymond Williams, Healer Practitioner Association International
Dr Ann Williamson
Daniel Wilson

Robert G Wood-Smith & Partners
World Health Organization
Dr Dominik Wujastyk
Yoga Biomedical Trust

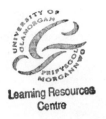

APPENDIX 9

Acronyms

AMRC	Association of Medical Research Charities
BMA	British Medical Association
CAM	Complementary and alternative medicine ("CAMs" is sometimes used as shorthand for "complementary and alternative therapies")
CHI	Commission for Health Improvement
CISCOM	Centralised Information Service for Complementary Medicine
CSM	Committee on Safety of Medicines
EMEA	European Agency for the Evaluation of Medicinal Products
ESCOP	European Scientific Cooperative on Phytotherapy
EU	European Union
FIM	Foundation for Integrated Medicine
GCC	General Chiropractic Council
GMC	General Medical Council
GOsC	General Osteopathic Council
GP	General Practitioner
HImP	Health Improvement Plan
MCA	Medicines Control Agency
MRC	Medical Research Council
NCCAM	US National Center for Complementary and Alternative Medicine
NHS	National Health Service
NICE	National Institute for Clinical Excellence
NIH	US National Institutes of Health
PAGB	Proprietary Association of Great Britain
PCG	Primary Care Group
PCT	Primary Care Trust
RCCM	Research Council for Complementary Medicine
RCT	Randomised Controlled Trial
R&D	Research and development
SSM	Special Study Module
TLC	Tender loving care
UKCC	UK Central Council for Nursing, Midwifery and Health Visiting
DNA	Deoxyribonucleic acid

Printed in the United Kingdom by The Stationery Office Limited
2/2001   597410   19585   CRC Supplied

ISBN 0-10-483100-6

9 780104 831007